Studies in Computational Intelligence

Volume 682

Series editor

Janusz Kacprzyk, Polish Academy of Sciences, Warsaw, Poland
e-mail: kacprzyk@ibspan.waw.pl

About this Series

The series "Studies in Computational Intelligence" (SCI) publishes new developments and advances in the various areas of computational intelligence—quickly and with a high quality. The intent is to cover the theory, applications, and design methods of computational intelligence, as embedded in the fields of engineering, computer science, physics and life sciences, as well as the methodologies behind them. The series contains monographs, lecture notes and edited volumes in computational intelligence spanning the areas of neural networks, connectionist systems, genetic algorithms, evolutionary computation, artificial intelligence, cellular automata, self-organizing systems, soft computing, fuzzy systems, and hybrid intelligent systems. Of particular value to both the contributors and the readership are the short publication timeframe and the worldwide distribution, which enable both wide and rapid dissemination of research output.

More information about this series at http://www.springer.com/series/7092

Robert Koprowski

Processing of Hyperspectral Medical Images

Applications in Dermatology Using MATLAB®

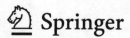 Springer

Robert Koprowski
Department of Biomedical Computer
   Systems, Institute of Computer Science
University of Silesia
Sosnowiec
Poland

Additional material to this book can be downloaded from http://extras.springer.com.

ISSN 1860-949X   ISSN 1860-9503   (electronic)
Studies in Computational Intelligence
ISBN 978-3-319-84410-7   ISBN 978-3-319-50490-2   (eBook)
DOI 10.1007/978-3-319-50490-2

® 2016 The MathWorks, Inc. MATLAB and Simulink are registered trade-marks of The MathWorks, Inc. See www.mathworks.com/trademarks for a list of additional trademarks. Other product or brand names may be trademarks or registered trademarks of their respective handles.

Printed on acid-free paper

This Springer imprint is published by Springer Nature
The registered company is Springer International Publishing AG
The registered company address is: Gewerbestrasse 11, 6330 Cham, Switzerland

Foreword

Medical imaging is a field of knowledge dealing with the methods of acquisition and analysis of images occurring in biological and medical research. The acquired images are used for research, diagnostic, therapeutic or educational purposes. The rapid development of diagnostic medical equipment and information technology enables the growing interaction of these two areas of expertise for the benefit of patients.

It is generally difficult to show the characteristics of real medical images pictorially and in a useful form for a physician. In addition to qualitative assessment, the physician also needs quantification of medical images, which will illustrate the various diagnostic parameters of medical objects. On their basis, the physician makes decisions related to the course of treatment, the strategy and the selection of appropriate drugs.

Quantitative assessment, achievable through the analysis of biomedical images, involves profiling contemporary analysis methods and algorithms. Such methods include not only image filtering but also its morphological and point transformations as well as their various classifications.

One of the rapidly developing techniques of image registration is the so-called hyperspectral imaging, which is used, inter alia, in biology and medicine. Issues related to the development of profiled software allowing for the hyperspectral analysis of biological and medical images is the goal of this monograph.

Zygmunt Wróbel

Preface

Modern methods of infrared, visible light or UV-light imaging are used in many fields of science, starting with astronomy through biophysics, physics, geography and ending with medicine. One such method allowing for imaging in a wide wavelength spectrum is hyperspectral imaging. The use of this type of imaging provides ample opportunities not only in terms of the qualitative assessment of acquired images but also in their quantification. The possibility of quantitative assessment is the result of analysis performed in the software provided with hyperspectral cameras. However, due to the large amount of data, this software has numerous limitations and is user-friendly in a limited way. On the other hand, there are well-known methods of 2D image analysis and processing. Their implementation in hyperspectral imaging is not an easy task. Apart from the need to extend 2D images into the third dimension (in which respect there are known methods of image analysis and processing, but in visible light), there remains the issue of optimization. It concerns optimization of computational complexity, optimization of analysis time and performance of preliminary calculations commonly used by users. The tasks that need to be solved by the users analysing hyperspectral medical images are also specific by their very nature. The specificity of these images stems directly from the inter-individual variability in patients and thus the images analysed. For this reason, for almost any task in question, object segmentation, comparison, calculation of characteristics, individual profiling of an algorithm are extremely important. Dedicated algorithms enable to conduct automated, repeatable measurements of, for example, a specific disease entity. However, profiled (dedicated) algorithms also have drawbacks—data overfitting. Therefore, these methods must be tested on images acquired under different conditions, with different hardware settings and for different operators, for example, a hyperspectral camera. Only in this case, it is certain that the proposed new algorithm will meet the requirements of universality when it comes to the data source and manner of acquisition and will be profiled for a particular application. Therefore, the key element is not only to propose new dedicated methods of hyperspectral image analysis and processing but also to try to implement them in practice and test their properties.

The presented methods of analysis and processing of hyperspectral medical images have been tested in practice in the Matlab® environment. The applied source code is attached to this monograph. The reader does not need to rewrite its fragments from the text. The source code is also described in detail in the monograph.

The monograph is intended for computer scientists, bioengineers, doctoral students and dermatologists interested in contemporary analysis methods. It can also be used to teach senior students of engineering studies related to computer science if the price of the book does not constitute a barrier. For the full understanding of the issues discussed, it has been assumed that the reader knows the basic methods and matrix operations in Matlab and knows the basic functions of Image Processing, Signal Processing and Statistics Toolboxes. Finally, other group of readers who want to know the way to solve the discussed problems in the field of image analysis and processing in Matlab may become interested in this monograph.

Sosnowiec, Poland   Robert Koprowski

Acknowledgments

First, I would like to thank Dr. Sławomir Wilczyński from the Medical University of Silesia in Katowice for the inspiration and consultations in the area of dermatological issues covered in the monograph. I would also like to thank Mr Raphael Stachiewicz from Enformatic Sp. z. o. o., Poland, for providing the hyperspectral camera. It allowed me to test the developed algorithms and perform measurements for objects other than medical ones.

I also thank Prof. Zygmunt Wróbel from the University of Silesia in Katowice, Poland, for his daily support and consultations.

Contents

Selected Symbols

m,u	Row
n,v	Column
i	Number of the image in a sequence—wavelength
$L(m,n,i)$	Point of the matrix of the image L
$L^{(C)}$	Image resulting from conditional operations
$L^{(D)}$	Image which complements the image L
L_{BIN}	Binary image
L_{GRAY}	Image in grey levels
$\ominus$	Erosion symbol
$\oplus$	Dilation symbol
$\rightarrow$	Neighbourhood type
h	Filter mask
p_r	Threshold
δ_g	Measurement error
σ	Standard deviation of the mean
θ	Angle of inclination of the filter
A	Amplitude
ACC	Accuracy
B	Number of bits of an image
FN	False negative
FP	False positive
I	Number of images in a sequence
M	Number of rows in a matrix
N	Number of columns in a matrix
SE	Structural element
SPC	Specificity
TN	True negative
TP	True positive
TPR	True positive rate

Chapter 1
Introduction

1.1 Purpose and Scope of the Monograph

The purpose of this monograph is to present new and known modified methods of hyperspectral image analysis and processing and profile them in terms of their usefulness in medical diagnostics and research, as well as develop quantitative diagnostic tools that can be used in everyday medical practice. The algorithms proposed in this monograph have the following characteristics:

- they are fully automatic—they do not require operator intervention, if it is necessary to provide additional parameters of the algorithm operation, they are selected automatically,
- the results obtained on their basis are fully reproducible,
- their operation was tested on a group of several thousands of hyperspectral images,
- they were implemented in Matlab,
- they have an open and tested source code attached to this monograph (in the form of an external link),
- they can be freely extended and modified—owing to the open source code.

The scope of the monograph includes medical images and, in particular, dermatological ones. However, they are only used to test the discussed methods. The scope of the monograph is divided into acquisition, image pre-processing, image processing and their classification presented in the following chapters.

© Springer International Publishing AG 2017
R. Koprowski, *Processing of Hyperspectral Medical Images*,
Studies in Computational Intelligence 682,
DOI 10.1007/978-3-319-50490-2_1

1.2 Material

Most of the images analysed in this monograph had a resolution $M \times N \times I = 696 \times 520 \times 128$, where M—the number of rows, N—the number of columns, I—the number of analysed wavelengths. Images of such or similar resolution (dependent on individual camera settings) were acquired with different hyperspectral cameras. The overwhelming part (approximately 75%) of all 200,000 images was registered using the SOC710-VP Hyperspectral Imager with a colour resolution $B = 12$ bits and spectral resolution from 400 to 1000 nm. This camera enables to register 128 bands ($I = 128$) and is powered by 12 V. The analysed images were obtained retrospectively and showed the skin of the hand, forearm, and other areas of the body recorded for dozens of patients. The patients were subject to exclusion criteria which were undisclosed skin diseases, fever, cardiac arrhythmias, seizures, inflammation of the skin and pregnancy. The analysed areas were illuminated by sunlight or using 40 W halogen lamps of a constant radiation spectrum ranging from 400 to 1000 nm. All the patients gave informed consent for the study which was conducted in accordance with the Declaration of Helsinki. No tests, measurements or experiments were performed on humans as part of this work. This monograph only deals with the methods of analysis of their images and diagnostic utility of the obtained results.

1.3 State of the Art

The subject of hyperspectral image analysis and the imaging method itself has been known for many years. On the day of writing this monograph, the end of 2016, the PubMed database contained 1922 publications containing the word "hyperspectral" in the title or description. Slightly different numbers (the number of articles) were given by the AuthorMapper database, namely 1825 publications, 18,643 authors from 6105 institutions. A breakdown by countries, institutions, authors, journals and subjects (the first 5 are listed) is presented in Table 1.1.

As shown above, the leaders in terms of publications on hyperspectral imaging are the United States, author Chang Chein-I and the area of Computer Science with 1420, 56, 1299 publications respectively. Image Processing and Computer Vision is a particularly exploited subject, which is extremely important from the point of view of this monograph. This subject includes such areas as (the number of publications is given in parentheses): Signal, Image and Video Processing (39); Journal of Real-Time Image Processing (37); Reference Recognition and Image Analysis (27); Hyperspectral Imaging (26); Real-Time Progressive Hyperspectral Image Processing (26); Neural Computing and Applications (25); Advances in Visual Computing (22) Image Analysis and Recognition (22); Image and Signal Processing (22); Multiple Classifier Systems (20); Machine Vision and Applications (19); Hyperspectral Data Compression (17); Advanced Concepts for

Table 1.1 The first 5 countries, 5 institutions, 5 authors, 5 journals, 5 subjects related to the word "hyperspectral"

Country	United States	China	Germany	India	France
Number of publications	1420 [1–5]	995 [6–10]	455 [11–15]	347 [16–20]	311 [21–25]
Institution	Chinese Academy of Sciences	Zhejiang University	University of California	University of Maryland	Wuhan University
Number of publications	162 [26–30]	67 [31–34]	64 [35–40]	47 [41–44]	43 [44–50]
Author	Chang, Chein-I [51, 52]	Graña, Manuel [53, 54]	Sun, Da-Wen [55–58]	Goodacre, Royston [59, 60]	Wang, Liguo [61, 62]
Number of publications	56	29	21	18	18
Journal	Precision Agriculture	Journal of the Indian Society of Remote Sensing	Environmental Monitoring and Assessment	Analytical and Bioanalytical Chemistry	Environmental Earth Sciences
Number of publications	144 [63, 64]	140 [65, 66]	100 [67, 68]	91 [69, 70]	77 [71, 72]
Subject	Computer Science	Life Sciences	Artificial Intelligence (incl. Robotics)	Earth Sciences	Image Processing and Computer Vision
Number of publications	1299 [73, 74]	960 [75, 76]	908 [77, 78]	859 [79, 80]	830 [81, 82]

Intelligent Vision Systems (16); Journal of Signal Processing Systems (16); Mathematical Morphology and Its Applications to Signal and Image Processing (15); Remote Sensing Digital Image Analysis (15); Image Analysis (14); Hyperspectral Image Fusion (13); Hyperspectral Image Processing (12); Journal of Mathematical Imaging and Vision (11).

When reviewing publications [83–91] in terms of the described research problems and their solutions, several open issues in the field of hyperspectral image analysis can be observed:

- the need for profiling methods of image analysis and processing to a particular research problem,
- lack of universal methods of analysis and
- lack of or limited availability of source codes.

Therefore, this monograph describes a sample application for the analysis and processing of hyperspectral images. The application was profiled to the area of biomedical engineering, and includes both known and new algorithms for image analysis and processing.

The discussed scope of biomedical engineering involves the use of hyperspectral cameras in dermatology. These issues have been partly presented in several publications [92–96]. Some of them are not profiled to solve a particular segmentation issue and do not address the issue of the algorithm sensitivity to parameter changes or the impact of different methods of acquisition on the results obtained. Accordingly, the analysis of the impact of acquisition on the results obtained, at the full automation of the proposed algorithm, constitutes another area (chapter) of this monograph.

1.4 Basic Definitions

Basic definitions apply to two issues:

- orientation of coordinate systems and
- assessment of the classifier quality.

They are described in the following sections.

1.4.1 Coordinate System

The orientation of the coordinate system is strongly dependent on the individual settings of the camera relative to the object, frame of reference. Regardless of the individual camera setting, to which all the described algorithms cannot be sensitive, it was assumed that the size of each image sequence would be defined by the number of rows M numbered from one, the number of columns N and the number of individual wavelengths I. The numbering from one and not zero, as in the case of well-known programming languages C++, C#, results from the adopted nomenclature and numbering in Matlab, Scilab or Octave. As a result, it was adopted in this monograph—Fig. 1.1 and Fig. 1.2.

The presented coordinate system (Fig. 1.1) will be used for all the presented analyses and algorithms. When an image (matrix) is a single 2D matrix, dimension I will be 1.

1.4.2 Evaluation of the Classifier Quality

Classifiers were usually induced by using the training data representing 2/3 of the total number of data. The remaining 1/3 of the data was used to test the classifier quality [96]. The training and test data were divided randomly. In the cases presented in this monograph, the division can be distorted. This is due to the fact that

Fig. 1.1 The following
symbols were adopted in the
coordinate system: *M* number
of rows, *N* number of
columns, *I* number of
wavelengths (random colours
of individual pixels were
adopted)

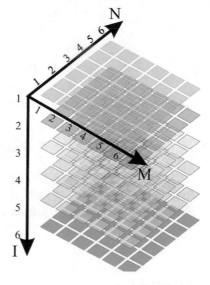

Fig. 1.2 Orientation of the
adopted coordinate system for
a colour image—RGB (pixel
colours correspond to R, G
and B components)

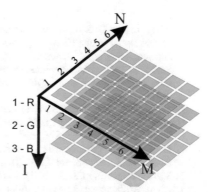

both the training and test vectors result from calculations for a sequence of images.
The number of images in the sequence to be analysed is affected by the operator.
Therefore, it does not have to be a strict division into 1/3 and 2/3. In each case,
evaluation of the classifier quality was based on determination of four values:

- **False Positive** (*FP*)—cases incorrectly classified as positive,
- **False Negative** (*FN*)—cases incorrectly classified as negative,
- **True Positive** (*TP*)—positive cases classified correctly,
- **True Negative** (*FN*)—negative cases classified correctly.

On their basis, sensitivity *TPR* and specificity *SPC* were defined as [97, 98]:

$$TPR = \frac{TP}{TP + FN} \cdot 100\% \tag{1.1}$$

$$SPC = \frac{TN}{TN + FP} \cdot 100\% \tag{1.2}$$

and accuracy ACC:

$$ACC = \frac{TP + TN}{TP + TN + FP + FN} \cdot 100\% \tag{1.3}$$

The parameters SPC and TPR will be the basis for creating the receiver operating characteristic curves (ROC), which are graphs of changes in TPR as a function of 100-SPC [99]. Additionally, the area under the curve (AUC) will be calculated [100].

References

1. Wang, Liguo; Zhao, Chunhui, Introduction of Hyperspectral Remote Sensing Applications, Hyperspectral Image Processing: 283–308, (2016).
2. Nguyen, Hien Van; Banerjee, Amit; Burlina, Philippe; Broadwater, Joshua; Chellappa, Rama, Tracking and Identification via Object Reflectance Using a Hyperspectral Video Camera, Machine Vision Beyond Visible Spectrum (2011-01-01) 1: 201–219, January 01, 2011.
3. Miguel, Agnieszka; Riskin, Eve; Ladner, Richard; Barney, Dane, Near-lossless and lossy compression of imaging spectrometer data: comparison of information extraction performance, Signal, Image and Video Processing (2012-11-01) 6: 597–611, November 01, 2012.
4. Le, Justin H.; Yazdanpanah, Ali Pour; Regentova, Emma E.; Muthukumar, Venkatesan A Deep Belief Network for Classifying Remotely-Sensed Hyperspectral Data, Advances in Visual Computing (2015-01-01): 9474, January 01, 2015.
5. Alam, Mohammad S.; Sakla, Adel Automatic Target Recognition in Multispectral and Hyperspectral Imagery Via Joint Transform Correlation, Wide Area Surveillance (2012-09-11) 6: 179–206, September 11, 2012.
6. Miller, Corey A.; Walls, Thomas J., Hyperspectral Scene Analysis via Structure from Motion, Advances in Visual Computing (2015-01-01): 9474, January 01, 2015.
7. Zou, Xiaobo; Zhao, Jiewen, Hyperspectral Imaging Detection, Nondestructive Measurement in Food and Agro-products (2015-01-01): 127–193, January 01, 2015.
8. Chen, Yu-Nan; Sun, Da-Wen; Cheng, Jun-Hu; Gao, Wen-Hong, Recent Advances for Rapid Identification of Chemical Information of Muscle Foods by Hyperspectral Imaging Analysis, Food Engineering Reviews (2016-04-04): 1–15, April 04, 2016.
9. Wang, Liguo; Zhao, Chunhui, Introduction of Hyperspectral Remote Sensing Applications, Hyperspectral Image Processing (2016-01-01): 283–308, January 01, 2016.
10. Zhang, Baohua; Fan, Shuxiang; Li, Jiangbo; Huang, Wenqian; Zhao, Chunjiang; Qian, Man; Zheng, Ling, Detection of Early Rottenness on Apples by Using Hyperspectral Imaging Combined with Spectral Analysis and Image Processing, Food Analytical Methods (2015-09-01) 8: 2075–2086, September 01, 2015.

11. Behmann, Jan; Mahlein, Anne-Katrin; Paulus, Stefan; Dupuis, Jan; Kuhlmann, Heiner; Oerke, Erich-Christian; Plümer, Lutz, Generation and application of hyperspectral 3D plant models: methods and challenges, Machine Vision and Applications (2015-10-03): 1–14, October 03, 2015.

12. Lausch, Angela; Pause, Marion; Merbach, Ines; Zacharias, Steffen; Doktor, Daniel; Volk, Martin; Seppelt, Ralf, A new multiscale approach for monitoring vegetation using remote sensing-based indicators in laboratory, field, and landscape, Environmental Monitoring and Assessment (2013-02-01) 185: 1215–1235, February 01, 2013.

13. Martin, Ron; Thies, Boris; Gerstner, Andreas OH, Hyperspectral hybrid method classification for detecting altered mucosa of the human larynx, International Journal of Health Geographics (2012-06-21) 11: 1–9, June 21, 2012.

14. Bigdeli, Behnaz; Samadzadegan, Farhad; Reinartz, Peter A Multiple SVM System for Classification of Hyperspectral Remote Sensing Data, Journal of the Indian Society of Remote Sensing (2013-12-01) 41: 763–776, December 01, 2013.

15. Wang, Ke; Gu, XingFa; Yu, Tao; Meng, QingYan; Zhao, LiMin; Feng, Li Classification of hyperspectral remote sensing images using frequency spectrum similarity, Science China Technological Sciences (2013-04-01) 56: 980–988, April 01, 2013.

16. Mookambiga, A.; Gomathi, V.Comprehensive review on fusion techniques for spatial information enhancement in hyperspectral imagery, Multidimensional Systems and Signal Processing (2016-04-27): 1–27, April 27, 2016.

17. Chutia, Dibyajyoti; Bhattacharyya, Dhruba Kumar; Kalita, Ranjan; Goswami, Jonali; Singh, Puyam S.; Sudhakar, S., A model on achieving higher performance in the classification of hyperspectral satellite data: a case study on Hyperion data, Applied Geomatics (2014-09-01) 6: 181–195, September 01, 2014.

18. Prabhu, N.; Arora, Manoj K.; Balasubramanian, R.Wavelet Based Feature Extraction Techniques of Hyperspectral Data, Journal of the Indian Society of Remote Sensing (2016-01-29): 1–12, January 29, 2016.

19. Prabhakar, M.; Prasad, Y. G.; Rao, Mahesh N., Remote Sensing of Biotic Stress in Crop Plants and Its Applications for Pest Management, Crop Stress and its Management: Perspectives and Strategies (2012-01-01): 517–545, January 01, 2012.

20. Vetrekar, N. T.; Gad, R. S.; Fernandes, I.; Parab, J. S.; Desai, A. R.; Pawar, J. D.; Naik, G. M.; Umapathy, S., Non-invasive hyperspectral imaging approach for fruit quality control application and classification: case study of apple, chikoo, guava fruits, Journal of Food Science and Technology (2015-11-01) 52: 6978–6989, November 01, 2015.

21. Licciardi, Giorgio Antonino Hyperspectral Data in Urban Areas Encyclopedia of Earthquake Engineering (2015-01-01): 1155–1164, January 01, 2015.

22. Luo, Bin; Chanussot, Jocelyn Supervised Hyperspectral Image Classification Based on Spectral Unmixing and Geometrical Features, Journal of Signal Processing Systems (2011-12-01) 65: 457–468, December 01, 2011.

23. Xia, Junshi; Chanussot, Jocelyn; Du, Peijun; He, Xiyan, Rotation-Based Ensemble Classifiers for High-Dimensional Data, Fusion in Computer Vision (2014-03-26): 135–160, March 26, 2014.

24. Hernández-Sánchez, Natalia; Moreda, Guillermo P.; Herre-ro-Langreo, Ana; Melado-Herreros, Ángela, Assessment of Internal and External Quality of Fruits and Vegetables, Imaging Technologies and Data Processing for Food Engineers (2016-01-01): 269–309, January 01, 2016.

25. Chen, Weishi; Guillaume, Mireille, HALS-based NMF with flexible constraints for hyperspectral unmixing, EURASIP Journal on Advances in Signal Processing (2012-03-05) 2012: 1–14, March 05, 2012.

26. Zhang, Bing; Yang, Wei; Gao, Lianru; Chen, Dongmei Real-time target detection in hyperspectral images based on spatial-spectral information extraction EURASIP Journal on Advances in Signal Processing (2012-07-13) 2012: 1–15, July 13, 2012.

27. Gao, Lianru; Zhang, Bing; Sun, Xu; Li, Shanshan; Du, Qian; Wu, Changshan Optimized maximum noise fraction for dimensionality reduction of Chinese HJ-1A hyperspectral data EURASIP Journal on Advances in Signal Processing (2013-04-02) 2013: 1–12, April 02, 2013.

28. Gao, Lianru; Zhuang, Lina; Wu, Yuanfeng; Sun, Xu; Zhang, Bing A quantitative and comparative analysis of different preprocessing implementations of DPSO: a robust endmember extraction algorithm Soft Computing (2014-11-06): 1–15, November 06, 2014.

29. Liu, Jun; Zhou, Xiran; Huang, Junyi; Liu, Shuguang; Li, Huali; Wen, Shan; Liu, Junchen Semantic classification for hyperspectral image by integrating distance measurement and relevance vector machine, Multimedia Systems (2015-03-18): 1–10, March 18, 2015.

30. Zhang, Hao; Hu, Hao; Zhang, Xiaobin; Wang, Kelin; Song, Tongqing; Zeng, Fuping Detecting Suaeda salsa L. chlorophyll fluorescence response to salinity stress by using hyperspectral reflectance, Acta Physiologiae Plantarum (2012-03-01) 34: 581–588, March 01, 2012.

31. Yu, Ke-Qiang; Zhao, Yan-Ru; Liu, Zi-Yi; Li, Xiao-Li; Liu, Fei; He, Yong Application of Visible and Near-Infrared Hyperspectral Imaging for Detection of Defective Features in Loquat Food and Bioprocess Technology (2014-11-01) 7: 3077–3087, November 01, 2014.

32. Li, Xiaorun; Cui, Jiantao; Zhao, Liaoying Blind nonlinear hyperspectral unmixing based on constrained kernel nonnegative matrix factorization, Signal, Image and Video Processing (2014-11-01) 8: 1555–1567, November 01, 2014.

33. Wu, Di; Wang, Songjing; Wang, Nanfei; Nie, Pengcheng; He, Yong; Sun, Da-Wen; Yao, Jiansong Application of Time Series Hyperspectral Imaging (TS-HSI) for Determining Water Distribution Within Beef and Spectral Kinetic Analysis During Dehydration Food and Bioprocess Technology (2013-11-01) 6: 2943–2958, November 01, 2013.

34. Pan, Leiqing; Lu, Renfu; Zhu, Qibing; Tu, Kang; Cen, Haiyan Predict Compositions and Mechanical Properties of Sugar Beet Using Hyperspectral Scattering, Food and Bioprocess Technology (2016-03-07): 1–10, March 07, 2016.

35. Martinelli, Federico; Scalenghe, Riccardo; Davino, Salvatore; Panno, Stefano; Scuderi, Giuseppe; Ruisi, Paolo; Villa, Paolo; Stroppiana, Daniela; Boschetti, Mirco; Goulart, Luiz R.; Davis, Cristina E.; Dandekar, Abhaya M. Advanced methods of plant disease detection. A review Agronomy for Sustainable Development (2015-01-01) 35: 1–25, January 01, 2015.

36. Khorram, Siamak; Koch, Frank H.; Wiele, Cynthia F.; Nelson, Stacy A. C.Data Acquisition Remote Sensing (2012-01-01): 17–37, January 01, 2012.

37. Pan, Zhihong; Healey, Glenn; Tromberg, Bruce Comparison of Spectral-Only and Spectral/Spatial Face Recognition for Personal Identity Verification EURASIP Journal on Advances in Signal Processing (2009-05-26) 2009: 1–6, May 26, 2009.

38. Underwood, E. C.; Mulitsch, M. J.; Greenberg, J. A.; Whiting, M. L.; Ustin, S. L.; Kefauver, S. C.Mapping Invasive Aquatic Vegetation in the Sacramento-San Joaquin Delta using Hyperspectral Imagery, Environmental Monitoring and Assessment (2006-10-01) 121: 47–64, October 01, 2006.

39. Herold, Martin; Roberts, Dar A. The Spectral Dimension in Urban Remote Sensing, Remote Sensing of Urban and Suburban Areas (2010-01-01) 10: 47–65, January 01, 2010.

40. Ramakrishna, Bharath; Plaza, Antonio J.; Chang, Chein-I; Ren, Hsuan; Du, Qian; Chang, Chein-Chi Spectral/Spatial Hyperspectral Image Compression, Hyperspectral Data Compression (2006-01-01): 309–346, January 01, 2006.

41. Benedetto, John J.; Czaja, Wojciech; Ehler, Martin Wavelet packets for time-frequency analysis of multispectral imagery, GEM - International Journal on Geomathematics (2013-11-01) 4: 137–154, November 01, 2013.

42. Yang, Chun-Chieh; Kim, Moon S.; Kang, Sukwon; Tao, Tao; Chao, Kuanglin; Lefcourt, Alan M.; Chan, Diane E. The development of a simple multispectral algorithm for detection of fecal contamination on apples using a hyperspectral line-scan imaging system, Sensing and Instrumentation for Food Quality and Safety (2011-03-01) 5: 10–18, March 01, 2011.

43. Safavi, Haleh; Chang, Chein-I; Plaza, Antonio J.Projection Pursuit-Based Dimensionality Reduction for Hyperspectral Analysis Satellite Data Compression (2011-01-01): 287–309, January 01, 2011.

44. Benedetto, John J.; Czaja, Wojciech Dimension Reduction and Remote Sensing Using Modern Harmonic Analysis, Handbook of Geomathematics (2015-01-01): 2609–2632, January 01, 2015.

45. Dian, Yuanyong; Fang, Shenghui; Le, Yuan; Xu, Yongrong; Yao, Chonghuai Comparison of the Different Classifiers in Vegetation Species Discrimination Using Hyperspectral Reflectance Data Journal of the Indian Society of Remote Sensing (2014-03-01) 42: 61–72, March 01,

46. Dian, Yuanyong; Le, Yuan; Fang, Shenghui; Xu, Yongrong; Yao, Chonghuai; Liu, Gang Influence of Spectral Bandwidth and Position on Chlorophyll Content Retrieval at Leaf and Canopy Levels Journal of the Indian Society of Remote Sensing (2016-02-13): 1–11, February 13, 2016.

47. Zhang, Liangpei; Zhong, Yanfei Analysis of Hyperspectral Remote Sensing Images Geospatial Technology for Earth Observation (2009-01-01): 235–269, January 01, 2009.

48. Du, Bo; Wang, Nan; Zhang, Liangpei; Tao, Dacheng Hyperspectral Medical Images Unmixing for Cancer Screening Based on Rotational Independent Component Analysis Intelligence Science and Big Data Engineering (2013-01-01) 8261: 336–343, January 01, 2013.

49. Zhang, Lefei; Zhang, Liangpei; Tao, Dacheng; Huang, Xin; Du, Bo Nonnegative Discriminative Manifold Learning for Hyperspectral Data Dimension Reduction Intelligence Science and Big Data Engineering (2013-01-01) 8261: 351–358, January 01, 2013.

50. Shen, Yingchun; Jin, Hai; Du, Bo An improved method to detect remote sensing image targets captured by sensor network Wuhan University Journal of Natural Sciences (2011-08-02) 16: 301–307, August 02, 2011.

51. Chang, Chein-I Hyperspectral Target Detection Real-Time Progressive Hyperspectral Image Processing (2016-01-01): 131–172, January 01, 2016.

52. Ramakrishna, Bharath; Plaza, Antonio J.; Chang, Chein-I; Ren, Hsuan; Du, Qian; Chang, Chein-Chi Spectral/Spatial Hyperspectral Image Compression, Hyperspectral Data Compression (2006-01-01): 309–346, January 01, 2006.

53. Veganzones, Miguel A.; Graña, Manuel Hybrid Computational Methods for Hyperspectral Image Analysis Hybrid Artificial Intelligent Systems (2012-01-01): 7209, January 01, 2012.

54. Moreno, Ramón; Graña, Manuel Segmentation of Hyperspectral Images by Tuned Chromatic Watershed Recent Advances in Knowledge-based Paradigms and Applications (2013-10-31) 234: 103–113, October 31, 2013.

55. Wu, Di; Sun, Da-Wen Hyperspectral Imaging Technology: A Nondestructive Tool for Food Quality and Safety Evaluation and Inspection Advances in Food Process Engineering Research and Applications (2013-09-13): 581–606, September 13, 2013.

56. Chen, Yu-Nan; Sun, Da-Wen; Cheng, Jun-Hu; Gao, Wen-Hong Recent Advances for Rapid Identification of Chemical Information of Muscle Foods by Hyperspectral Imaging Analysis Food Engineering Reviews (2016-04-04): 1–15, April 04, 2016.

57. Wu, Di; Sun, Da-Wen Hyperspectral Imaging Technology: A Nondestructive Tool for Food Quality and Safety Evaluation and Inspection Advances in Food Process Engineering Research and Applications (2013-09-13): 581–606, September 13, 2013.

58. Chen, Yu-Nan; Sun, Da-Wen; Cheng, Jun-Hu; Gao, Wen-Hong Recent Advances for Rapid Identification of Chemical Information of Muscle Foods by Hyperspectral Imaging Analysis Food Engineering Reviews (2016-04-04): 1–15, April 04, 2016.

59. Goodacre, Royston; Burton, Rebecca; Kaderbhai, Naheed; Timmins, Éadaoin M.; Woodward, Andrew; Rooney, Paul J.; Kell, Douglas B. Intelligent Systems for the Characterization of Microorganisms from Hyperspectral Data Rapid Methods for Analysis of Biological Materials in the Environment (2000-01-01) 30: 111–136, January 01, 2000.

60. Winder, Catherine L.; Cornmell, Robert; Schuler, Stephanie; Jarvis, Roger M.; Stephens, Gill M.; Goodacre, Royston Metabolic fingerprinting as a tool to monitor whole-cell biotransformations Analytical and Bioanalytical Chemistry (2011-01-01) 399: 387-401, January 01, 2011.
61. Wang, Liguo; Zhao, Chunhui Introduction of Hyperspectral Remote Sensing Applications Hyperspectral Image Processing (2016-01-01): 283-308, January 01, 2016.
62. Yang, Jinghui; Wang, Liguo; Qian, Jinxi Hyperspectral Imagery Classification Based on Sparse Feature and Neighborhood Homogeneity, Journal of the Indian Society of Remote Sensing (2015-09-01) 43: 445-457, September 01, 2015.
63. Yang, Chenghai; Everitt, James H. Using spectral distance, spectral angle and plant abundance derived from hyperspectral imagery to characterize crop yield variation, Precision Agriculture (2012-02-01) 13: 62-75, February 01, 2012.
64. Yang, Chenghai; Everitt, James H.; Bradford, Joe M. Airborne hyperspectral imagery and linear spectral unmixing for mapping variation in crop yield, Precision Agriculture (2007-12-01) 8: 279-296, December 01, 2007.
65. Prabhu, N.; Arora, Manoj K.; Balasubramanian, R. Wavelet Based Feature Extraction Techniques of Hyperspectral Data, Journal of the Indian Society of Remote Sensing (2016-01-29): 1–12, January 29, 2016.
66. Yang, Jinghui; Wang, Liguo; Qian, Jinxi Hyperspectral Imagery Classification Based on Sparse Feature and Neighborhood Homogeneity, Journal of the Indian Society of Remote Sensing (2015-09-01) 43: 445–457, September 01, 2015.
67. Lausch, Angela; Pause, Marion; Merbach, Ines; Zacharias, Steffen; Doktor, Daniel; Volk, Martin; Seppelt, Ralf A new multiscale approach for monitoring vegetation using remote sensing-based indicators in laboratory, field, and landscape Environmental Monitoring and Assessment (2013-02-01) 185: 1215–1235, February 01, 2013.
68. Lausch, Angela; Pause, Marion; Doktor, Daniel; Preidl, Sebastian; Schulz, Karsten Monitoring and assessing of landscape heterogeneity at different scales Environmental Monitoring and Assessment (2013-11-01) 185: 9419–9434, November 01, 2013.
69. Vermeulen, Ph.; Fernández Pierna, J. A.; Egmond, H. P.; Zegers, J.; Dardenne, P.; Baeten, V.Validation and transferability study of a method based on near-infrared hyperspectral imaging for the detection and quantification of ergot bodies in cereals Analytical and Bioanalytical Chemistry (2013-09-01) 405: 7765–7772, September 01, 2013.
70. Williams, Paul J.; Geladi, Paul; Britz, Trevor J.; Manley, Marena Near-infrared (NIR) hyperspectral imaging and multivariate image analysis to study growth characteristics and differences between species and strains of members of the genus Fusarium Analytical and Bioanalytical Chemistry (2012-10-01) 404: 1759–1769, October 01, 2012.
71. Ebadi, Ladan; Shafri, Helmi Z. M.; Mansor, Shattri B.; Ashurov, Ravshan A review of applying second-generation wavelets for noise removal from remote sensing data Environmental Earth Sciences (2013-11-01) 70: 2679–2690, November 01, 2013.
72. Ebadi, Ladan; Shafri, Helmi Z. M.Compression of remote sensing data using second-generation wavelets: a review Environmental Earth Sciences (2014-02-01) 71: 1379–1387, February 01, 2014.
73. Veganzones, Miguel A.; Graña, Manuel Hybrid Computational Methods for Hyperspectral Image Analysis Hybrid Artificial Intelligent Systems (2012-01-01): 7209, January 01, 2012.
74. Qian, Shen-En Development of On-Board Data Compression Technology at Canadian Space Agency Satellite Data Compression (2011-01-01): 1–28, January 01, 2011.
75. Zou, Xiaobo; Zhao, Jiewen Hyperspectral Imaging Detection Nondestructive Measurement in Food and Agro-products (2015-01-01): 127–193, January 01, 2015.
76. Prabhakar, M.; Prasad, Y. G.; Rao, Mahesh N. Remote Sensing of Biotic Stress in Crop Plants and Its Applications for Pest Management Crop Stress and its Management: Perspectives and Strategies (2012-01-01): 517–545, January 01, 2012.
77. Mookambiga, A.; Gomathi, V. Comprehensive review on fusion techniques for spatial information enhancement in hyperspectral imagery, Multidimensional Systems and Signal Processing (2016-04-27): 1–27, April 27, 2016.

78. Appice, Annalisa; Guccione, Pietro; Malerba, Donato Transductive hyperspectral image classification: toward integrating spectral and relational features via an iterative ensemble system Machine Learning (2016-03-22): 1–33, March 22, 2016.

79. Prabhu, N.; Arora, Manoj K.; Balasubramanian, R. Wavelet Based Feature Extraction Techniques of Hyperspectral Data, Journal of the Indian Society of Remote Sensing (2016-01-29): 1–12, January 29, 2016.

80. Hasanlou, Mahdi; Samadzadegan, Farhad; Homayouni, Saeid SVM-based hyperspectral image classification using intrinsic dimension Arabian Journal of Geosciences (2015-01-01) 8: 477–487, January 01, 2015.

81. Chang, Chein-I Back Matter - Real-Time Progressive Hyperspectral Image Processing Real-Time Progressive Hyperspectral Image Processing (2016-01-01), January 01, 2016.

82. Wang, Liguo; Zhao, Chunhui Introduction of Hyperspectral Remote Sensing Applications Hyperspectral Image Processing (2016-01-01): 283–308, January 01, 2016.

83. Chaudhuri, Subhasis; Kotwal, Ketan Introduction Hyperspectral Image Fusion (2013-01-01): 1–18, January 01, 2013.

84. Wang, Liguo; Zhao, Chunhui Basic Theory and Main Processing Techniques of Hyperspectral Remote Sensing Hyperspectral Image Processing (2016-01-01): 1–44, January 01, 2016.

85. Ülkü, İrem; Töreyin, Behçet Uğur Sparse coding of hyperspectral imagery using online learning Signal, Image and Video Processing (2015-05-01) 9: 959–966, May 01, 2015.

86. Sánchez, Sergio; Plaza, Antonio Fast determination of the number of endmembers for real-time hyperspectral unmixing on GPUs Journal of Real-Time Image Processing (2014-09-01) 9: 397–405, September 01, 2014.

87. Li, Xiaorun; Cui, Jiantao; Zhao, Liaoying Blind nonlinear hyperspectral unmixing based on constrained kernel nonnegative matrix factorization Signal, Image and Video Processing (2014-11-01) 8: 1555–1567, November 01, 2014.

88. Qin, Zhen; Shi, Zhenwei; Jiang, Zhiguo A quasi-Newton-based spatial multiple materials detector for hyperspectral imagery Neural Computing and Applications (2013-08-01) 23: 403–409, August 01, 2013.

89. Chang, Chein-I Hyperspectral Target Detection Real-Time Progressive Hyperspectral Image Processing (2016-01-01): 131–172, January 01, 2016.

90. Luo, Bin; Chanussot, Jocelyn Supervised Hyperspectral Image Classification Based on Spectral Unmixing and Geometrical Features Journal of Signal Processing Systems (2011-12-01) 65: 457–468, December 01, 2011.

91. Wang, Tao; Zhu, Zhigang; Krzaczek, Robert S.; Rhody, Harvey E. A System Approach to Adaptive Multimodal Sensor Designs Machine Vision Beyond Visible Spectrum (2011-01-01) 1: 159–176, January 01, 2011.

92. Shao, Ming; Wang, Yunhong; Liu, Peijiang Face Relighting Based on Multi-spectral Quotient Image and Illumination Tensorfaces Computer Vision – ACCV 2009 (2010-01-01) 5996: 108–117, January 01, 2010.

93. Fadzil, M. H. Ahmad; Nugroho, Hermawan; Jolivot, Romuald; Marzani, Franck; Shamsuddin, Norashikin; Baba, Roshidah Modelling of Reflectance Spectra of Skin Phototypes III Visual Informatics: Sustaining Research and Innovations (2011-01-01) 7066: 352–360, January 01, 2011.

94. Lefèvre, Sébastien; Aptoula, Erchan; Perret, Benjamin; Weber, Jonathan Morphological Template Matching in Color Images Advances in Low-Level Color Image Processing (2013-12-17) 11: 241–277, December 17, 2013.

95. Galeano, July; Jolivot, Romuald; Marzani, Franck Analysis of Human Skin Hyper-Spectral Images by Non-negative Matrix Factorization Advances in Soft Computing (2011-01-01) 7095: 431–442, January 01, 2011.

96. Jia, Hongjie; Ding, Shifei; Meng, Lingheng; Fan, Shuyan A density-adaptive affinity propagation clustering algorithm based on spectral dimension reduction Neural Computing and Applications (2014-12-01) 25: 1557–1567, December 01, 2014.

97. Fisher R. A. The Use of Multiple Measurements in Taxonomic Problems, Annals of Eugenics, 1936, 7, 179–88.
98. Hanley J.A., McNeil B. J., The meaning and use of the area under receiving operating characteristic (ROC) curve, Radiology 1982, 43, 29–36.
99. Anscombe F. J., Graphs in Statistical Analysis, The American Statistician, 27 (1973), 17–21.
100. Bradley A. P., The use of the area under the ROC curve in the evaluation of machine learning algorithms, Reference Recognition, 1997, 30 (7), 1145–59.

Chapter 2
Image Acquisition

2.1 Introduction

Image acquisition was carried out with the SOC710-VP hyperspectral camera. The camera was positioned perpendicular to the table on which the object was placed. The scanning area and the focal length were selected in such a way that the analysed object filled, if possible, the entire stage—Fig. 2.1.

Two different types of illumination were adopted:

- natural light—sunlight,
- artificial lighting—40 W halogen lamps with a constant radiation spectrum in the range from 400 to 1000 nm.

For each registered image $L_{GRAY}(m, n, i)$, a reference gray level in the full spectrum sized 10 cm × 10 cm was used as a reference—Fig. 2.2. The reference was an integral part of the camera equipment. In addition, for testing purposes, for several cases, two additional series of images were recorded when there was no light $L_{DARK}(m, n, i)$ and for the full illumination $L_{WHITE}(m, n, i)$—in both cases without an object. The images $L_{DARK}(m, n, i)$, $L_{WHITE}(m, n, i)$ are the basis for normalization of the image $L_{GRAY}(m, n, i)$ which is described in the next chapter.

All images are saved in a *.cube format. They can also be saved in other formats, *.raw and *.dat, which are further converted to Matlab in the form of a three-dimensional matrix [1]. This conversion is specific to each of these types of record (*.cube, *.raw or *.dat). The files with these extensions are saved by the hyperspectral camera in the format shown in Fig. 2.3.

Saving data in the hyperspectral camera stems from the idea of its operation. The first data saved to *.cube, *.raw or *.dat * files relate to the first row or column (depending on the camera position relative to the object). The first row is stored for all the wavelengths $i \in (1, I)$, then the next row etc. The number of rows, columns

© Springer International Publishing AG 2017
R. Koprowski, *Processing of Hyperspectral Medical Images*,
Studies in Computational Intelligence 682,
DOI 10.1007/978-3-319-50490-2_2

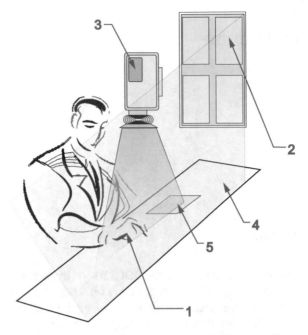

Fig. 2.1 Image acquisition—the position of the camera relative to the subject: *1* test object—hand; *2* window; *3* hyperspectral camera; *4* table top illuminated by sunlight; *5* reference

Fig. 2.2 Zoom of the acquisition area for artificial lighting: *1* test object—subject's hand; *2* grey reference; *3* stage; *4* halogen bulbs

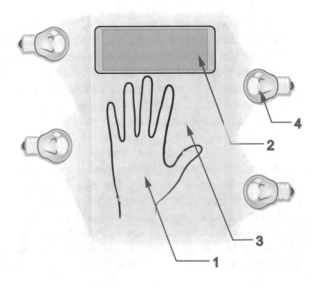

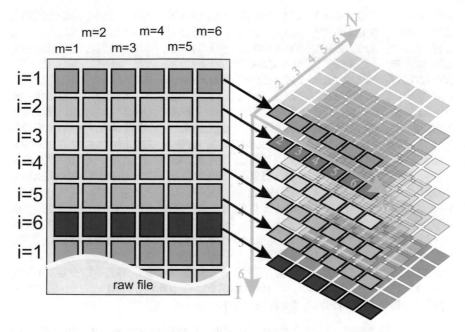

Fig. 2.3 Data organization in **.raw*, **.cube* and **.dat* files

and individual wavelengths is stored in a separate **.hdr* file. An example of its
structure is shown below:

ENVI
Description = {}
samples = 520
lines = 696
bands = 128
header offset = 32768
major frame offsets = {0, 0}
file type = ENVI Standard
data type = 12
interleave = bil
sensor type = Unknown
byte order = 0
wavelength units = Unknown
wavelength = {
374.980011, 379.953130, 384.929945, 389.910456, 394.894663, 399.882566,
404.874165, 409.869460, 414.868451, 419.871138, 424.877521, 429.887600,
434.901375, 439.918846, 444.940014, 449.964877, 454.993436, 460.025691,

465.061642, 470.101289, 475.144632, 480.191671, 485.242406, 490.296837, 495.354964, 500.416787, 505.482306, 510.551521, 515.624432, 520.701039, 525.781342, 530.865341, 535.953036, 541.044427, 546.139514, 551.238297, 556.340776, 561.446951, 566.556822, 571.670389, 576.787652, 581.908612, 587.033267, 592.161618, 597.293665, 602.429408, 607.568847, 612.711982, 617.858813, 623.009340, 628.163563, 633.321482, 638.483097, 643.648408, 648.817415, 653.990118, 659.166517, 664.346612, 669.530403, 674.717890, 679.909073, 685.103952, 690.302527, 695.504798, 700.710765, 705.920428, 711.133787, 716.350842, 721.571594, 726.796041, 732.024184, 737.256023, 742.491558, 747.730789, 752.973716, 758.220339, 763.470658, 768.724673, 773.982384, 779.243791, 784.508894, 789.777693, 795.050188, 800.326379, 805.606266, 810.889849, 816.177128, 821.468103, 826.762774, 832.061141, 837.363204, 842.668963, 847.978418, 853.291569, 858.608416, 863.928959, 869.253199, 874.581134, 879.912765, 885.248092, 890.587115, 895.929834, 901.276249, 906.626360, 911.980167, 917.337670, 922.698869, 928.063764, 933.432355, 938.804642, 944.180625, 949.560304, 954.943679, 960.330750, 965.721517, 971.115980, 976.514139, 981.915994, 987.321545, 992.730792, 998.143735,   1003.560374,   1008.980709,   1014.404740,   1019.832467, 1025.263891, 1030.699010, 1036.137825}

The arrangement of individual elements is typical for almost all types of hyperspectral cameras. The first elements of the header are designed to provide information on the number of samples (*samples = 520*) or the number of columns *N*, then the number of lines (*lines = 696*) or the number of rows *M* and the number of different wavelengths (*bands = 128*) or *I*-th number of a matrix sized $M \times N$. Then there are two more important elements: header offset = 32,768 relating to the transfer of data in bytes (in this case 32,768 bytes), and data type *data type = 12* meaning that there is 16-bit unsigned integer per one pixel [2]. For other values of variable '*data type*' per one pixel there is:

- 8-bit unsigned integer (*data type = 1*),
- 16-bit signed integer (*data type = 2*),
- 32-bit signed integer (*data type = 3*),
- 32-bit single-precision (*data type = 4*),
- 64-bit double-precision floating-point (*data type = 5*),
- real-imaginary pair of single-precision floating-point (*data type = 6*),
- 16-bit unsigned integer (*data type = 12*),
- 32-bit unsigned long integer (*data type = 13*),
- 64-bit long integer (*data type = 14*),
- 64-bit unsigned long integer (*data type = 15*).

The last element in the *.hdr* file is the variable *wavelength*. It means the wavelengths in nanometres for which the individual images were acquired. In the present case, it is 374.980011 nm ($i = 1$), 379.953130 nm ($i = 2$), 384.929945 nm ($i = 3$) etc.

Therefore, the *.hdr* file is useful as it downloads the parameters (number of rows, columns, wavelengths) necessary to read data in the *.cube*, *.raw* or *.dat* files. The following are excerpts (separated by '...') of the source code of the file read_envi_header enabling to read and interpret the file *.hdr* consisting of three blocks: the search for the sign ' { } = ', the search for the numerical value of the variable lines and the values of the variable 'Wavelength' i.e.:

```
function
[lines,bands,samples,Wavelength,data_type,header_offse
t]=read_envi_header(src)

. . .

fid = fopen(src);
[drep] = textscan(fid,'%s','delimiter','{}=
','MultipleDelimsAsOne', 1);
fclose(fid); drep_=drep{:,1};

Dlines=strcmpi(drep{1,:},'lines');
DlinesY=[Dlines,(1:size(Dlines,1))'];
DlinesY(DlinesY(:,1)~=1,:)=[];
nrl=DlinesY(1,2);
lines=str2num(str2mat(drep_{nrl+1}));

. . .

Dwavelength=strcmpi(drep{1,:},'Wavelength');
DwavelengthY=[Dwavelength,(1:size(Dwavelength,1))'];
DwavelengthY(DwavelengthY(:,1)~=1,:)=[];
nrsw=DwavelengthY(end,2);
Wavelength=str2num(str2mat(drep_{(nrsw+1)  :
(nrsw+1+bands-1)}));

. . .
```

The dots '...' (as mentioned above) mean that some part of the source code has been removed. It should be noted that they play a different role than the dotted line '...' in Matlab which indicates that a further part of the code will be continued in the next line.

The read values of lines, bands, samples, Wavelength, data_type, header_offset are further used for reading the image data contained in the files *.*cube*, *.*raw* or *.*dat*. The function designed for this purpose called read_envi_-data is as follows:

```
function
[LGRAY]=read_envi_data(src,lines,bands,samples,data_ty
pe,band_no,header_offset)

...

if (data_type~=12) && (data_type~=4)
    disp('Unsupported file type')
else
    fid = fopen(src);
    frewind(fid)
    if data_type==12
        fseek(fid,band_no*samples*2+header_offset,
'bof');
        [LGRAY, COUNT] =
fread(fid,[samples,lines],[mat2str(samples),'*integer*
2'],samples*bands*2-samples*2);
    else % data_type==4
        fseek(fid,band_no*samples*4+header_offset,
'bof');
        [LGRAY, COUNT] =
fread(fid,[samples,lines],[mat2str(samples),'*float'],
samples*bands*4-samples*4);
    end
    fclose(fid);
    LGRAY=LGRAY';
end
```

In its first part, the data type is checked. Two types of data mentioned above numbered '12' and '4' are handled [3]. If the data type is different, the message 'Unsupported file type' will be displayed. Then the data will be read from the header_offset. The reading for the data type '12' takes place every samples*bands*2-samples*2 while in the case of data type '4' every samples*bands*4-samples*4, 16 and 32 bits per pixel respectively. The result is the matrix L_{GRAY} used for image pre-processing.

References

1. Robert Koprowski, Sławomir Wilczyński, Zygmunt Wróbel, Barbara Błońska-Fajfrowska, Calibration and segmentation of skin areas in hyperspectral imaging for the needs of dermatology, BioMedical Engineering OnLine 2014 13:113.
2. Koprowski R, Wilczyński S, Wróbel Z, Kasperczyk S, Błońska-Fajfrowska B. Automatic method for the dermatological diagnosis of selected hand skin features in hyperspectral imaging. Biomed Eng Online. 2014 13:47.
3. Koprowski R. Hyperspectral imaging in medicine: image pre-processing problems and solutions in Matlab. J Biophotonics. 2015 Nov;8(11–12):935–43. doi: 10.1002/jbio. 201400133. Epub 2015 Feb 9.

Chapter 3
Image Pre-Processing

Preliminary analysis and processing of images is associated with three main elements:

- affine transformation of the image,
- image filtering and
- image calibration.

These three elements are presented in the following subchapters. The source code of these three elements was implemented in three Matlab files: GUI_hyperspectral_trans, GUI_hyperspectral and GUI_hyperspectral_fun. The first one concerns affine transformations, the second one relates to the graphical user interface and the third one concerns the function associated with the response to specific user's actions. The content, source code, of these functions (mainly GUI_hyperspectral_fun) will be presented in fragments in the order of its description in the text.

It is possible to read the image owing to the functions read_envi_data and read_envi_header described above. In the file GUI_hyperspectral_fun, each 2D image read correctly is saved to disk with the same name as the input file *.cube, *.raw or *.dat with the extension *.mat. When re-reading the file *.cube, *.raw or *.dat, it is checked whether the file *.mat exists. If it exists, it is loaded. Saving individual 2D files with the extension *.mat means that the data are read at least 2 times faster. A fragment of the source code of the file GUI_hyperspectral_fun is shown below:

© Springer International Publishing AG 2017
R. Koprowski, *Processing of Hyperspectral Medical Images*,
Studies in Computational Intelligence 682,
DOI 10.1007/978-3-319-50490-2_3

```
try
    load([src,mat2str(band_no),'.mat'],'L1');
catch
[L1]=read_envi_data(src,lines,bands,samples,data_type,
band_no,header_offset);
    save([src,mat2str(band_no),'.mat'],'L1');
    L_(:,band_no,[1 3])=0;L_(:,band_no,2)=1;
end
```

The menu allowing for the selection of the file *.cube, *.raw or *.dat is invoked at the beginning of the function GUI_hyperspectral_fun, i.e.:

```
[FileName,PathName,FilterIndex] = uiget-
file({'*.cube';'*.dat';'*.raw'},'Select file');
if FilterIndex~=0
    src=[PathName,FileName];
    if strcmp(src(end-2:end),'ube')
[lines,bands,samples,Wavelength,data_type,header_offse
t]=read_envi_header([src(1:end-4),'hdr']);
    else
[lines,bands,samples,Wavelength,data_type,header_offse
t]=read_envi_header([src(1:end-3),'hdr']);
    end
band_no=round(bands/2);
[L1]=read_envi_data(src,lines,bands,samples,data_type,
band_no,header_offset);
```

According to the source code shown above, the middle 2D image from the image sequence, when properly loaded, is displayed by default. Since the number of individual *.mat files initially converted by Matlab (with prior reading of the same file) is not known, its status is read. Reading and showing the status in the visual form involves a sequential attempt to read all the files *.mat, i.e.:

```
L_=cat(3,ones([20 bands]),zeros([20 bands]),zeros([20
bands]));
          for band_no=1:bands
              if ex-
ist([src,mat2str(band_no),'.mat'])==2
                  L_(:,band_no,[1
3])=0;L_(:,band_no,2)=1;
                  end
          end
        Lvar=imresize(L_,[20 800]);
Lvar(Lvar<0)=0;Lvar(Lvar>1)=1;
        set(hObj(20),'CData',Lvar);
```

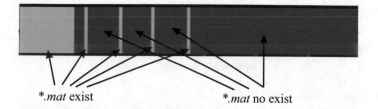

*.mat exist   *.mat no exist

Fig. 3.1 Exemplary image indicating the distribution: the existence of the file *.mat is shown in *green*, its absence in *red*

The displayed image is 20 × 800 pixels. The red stripes represent the absence of the *.mat file, while the green ones mean that it is located on the disk. An exemplary image is shown in Fig. 3.1.

3.1 Affine Transformations of the Image

The range of affine transformations applied in hyperspectral imaging is much wider than in the case of classic 2D images. Only those which are most often applied in hyperspectral imaging were selected. These are:

- rotation by any angle in the angular range of $\alpha \in (0,360]$ degrees every 10 degrees—the new coordinates of pixels in this case (m_A, n_A) are as follows:

$$n_A = \frac{N}{2} + \left(n - \frac{N}{2}\right) \cdot \cos(\alpha) - \left(m - \frac{M}{2}\right) \cdot \sin(\alpha) \qquad (3.1)$$

$$m_A = \frac{M}{2} + \left(n - \frac{N}{2}\right) \cdot \sin(\alpha) + \left(m - \frac{M}{2}\right) \cdot \cos(\alpha) \qquad (3.2)$$

- reordering of rows—the image $L_{GRAYM}(m, n, i)$—mirrored around the x-axis,
- reordering of columns—the image $L_{GRAYN}(m, n, i)$—mirrored around the y-axis, i.e.:

$$L_{GRAYM}(m, n, i) = L_{GRAY}(M - m, n, i) \qquad (3.3)$$

$$L_{GRAYN}(m, n, i) = L_{GRAY}(m, N - n, i) \qquad (3.4)$$

- Cropping—cutting a portion of the image, i.e.:

$$L_{GRAYROI} = L_{GRAY}(m, n, i) \qquad\qquad (3.5)$$

where: $m, n \in ROI$.

Since in practice, the user manually selects the option of rotation, shift or cropping, the variable names in the function were standardized to 'L1' for simplicity. In practice, a record in the source code overwrites the value in variable $L1$, but it is consistent and clear:

```
if get(hObj(7),'Value')==1 % ROI
if min(r(2:3))>1
    L1=L1(r(2):(r(2)+r(4)),r(1):(r(1)+r(3)));
end
end

if get(hObj(8),'Value')==1
    L1=L1(:,end:-1:1);
end
if get(hObj(9),'Value')==1
    L1=L1(end:-1:1,:);
end
if get(hObj(10),'Value')==1
    L1=mat2gray(L1);
end
if get(hObj(12),'Value')~=1
    L1=imrotate(L1,(get(hObj(12),'Value')-
1)*10,'crop');
end
```

For each condition `if`, the value set by the user is taken—from the handle `hObj`. In this case, these are the handles to `checkbox` (7,8,9,10) and the pull-down menu (`popup`), the value of 12.

3.2   Image Filtration

3.2.1   Non-Adaptive

The read image $L_{GRAY}(m, n, i)$ and the calibrated images $L_{DARK}(m, n, i)$ and $L_{WHITE}(m, n, i)$ are subjected to noise removal. The noise is removed using a median filter with a mask h_w sized $M_w \times N_w = 3 \times 3$ pixels or more set manually using the graphical user interface (GUI). Each 2D image is filtered individually. The minimum size of the mask h_w was selected based on the maximum size of a single distortion whose area of concentration did not exceed 4 pixels. The size of distortions in hyperspectral images may be different and therefore the size of the filter is set manually. The specific size is set in the menu checkbox with the handle hObj(14), i.e.:

```
if get(hObj(14),'Value')==2
    L1=medfilt2(L1,[3 3],'symmetric');
end
if get(hObj(14),'Value')==3
    L1=medfilt2(L1,[5 5],'symmetric');
end
if get(hObj(14),'Value')==4
    L1=medfilt2(L1,[7 7],'symmetric');
end
if get(hObj(14),'Value')==5
    L1=medfilt2(L1,[9 9],'symmetric');
end
if get(hObj(14),'Value')==6
    L1=medfilt2(L1,[11 11],'symmetric');
end
```

The above source code shows that for the value '1', the image $L1$ is not filtered in any way, and the filtration itself ranges from $M_w \times N_w = 3 \times 3$ pixels to $M_w \times N_w = 11 \times 11$ pixels. This is enough to remove noise from most hyperspectral images.

3.2.2 Adaptive

The second type of noise removal from a sequence of hyperspectral images is adaptive adjustment of the size of the filter [1–7], for example, the median filter. There are three options here:

- adaptation of the filter size to the 2D image content independently for each i-th image,
- adaptation to the i-th 2D image—depending on the wavelength,
- adaptation of the filter size to both the 2D image content and the i-th image.

Choosing the right solution for hyperspectral images should be preceded by the analysis of changes in the Peak Signal-to-Noise Ratio (PSNR) for individual i images in a series of measurements. The values of PSNR, the vector $L_{PSNR}(i)$, are defined as:

$$L_{PSNR}(i) = 10 \cdot \log_{10}\left(\frac{(2^B - 1)^2}{L_{MSE}(m, n, i)}\right) \tag{3.6}$$

where: B is the number of bits per one image pixel, $L_{MSE}(m, n, i)$ is the mean squared error. i.e.:

$$L_{MSE}(m, n, i) = \frac{1}{M \cdot N} \sum_{m=1}^{M} \sum_{n=1}^{N} (L_{MEAN}(i) - L_{GRAY}(m, n, i))^2 \qquad (3.7)$$

$$L_{MEAN}(i) = \frac{1}{M \cdot N} \sum_{m=1}^{M} \sum_{n=1}^{N} L_{GRAY}(m, n, i) \qquad (3.8)$$

The problem of selecting the size of the filter h_w (its size $M_w \times N_w$) and making it dependent on $L_{PSNR}(i)$ is directly related to the content of images. This content may be different in each case—especially when it comes to diagnosis of the skin. In this regard, the selected *ROIs* shown in Fig. 3.2 were analysed.

The sample results shown in Fig. 3.2 confirm an increase in noise for hyperspectral cameras for extreme wavelength values. In addition, it should be noted that median filtering with a mask h_w sized 3×3 pixels increases the value of PSNR to the greatest extent (almost 10 dB). The source code of *m-file* GUI_hyperspectral_filter_test providing the above graphs is as follows:

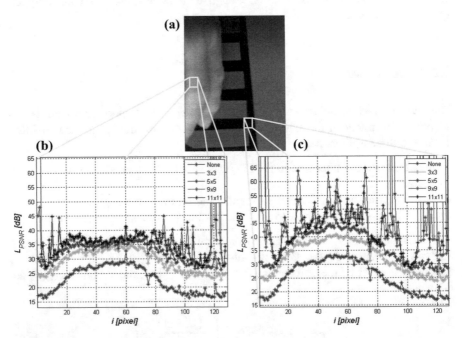

Fig. 3.2 Results of analysis of PSNR values for two selected regions: **a** the input image $L_{GRAY}(m, n, i = 80)$, **b** a graph of changes in $L_{PSNR}(i)$ for i images without median filtering and with median filtering using masks sized $M_w \times N_w = 3 \times 3$, 5×5, 9×9 and 11×11 pixels; **c** an analogous graph for another *ROI*

```
L1=load(['D:/k/_I20_L0-511_13-1-
2016_13.5.59.cube',mat2str(80),'.mat']);
Lgrayi=mat2gray(L1.L1);
figure;
[X,Y,I2,RECT] = IMCROP(Lgrayi);
hObj=waitbar(0,'Please wait...');
LPSNR=[];
for i=1:128
    L1=load(['D:/k/_I20_L0-511_13-1-
2016_13.5.59.cube',mat2str(i),'.mat']);
    Lgrayi=mat2gray(L1.L1);
    Lgrayi=IMCROP(Lgrayi,RECT);
    LPSNR(i,1)=20*log10(1)-10*log10( sum(sum(
(mean(Lgrayi(:)) - Lgrayi).^2 )) ./ (size(Lgrayi,1) *
size(Lgrayi,2)) );

    Lgrayi=mat2gray(L1.L1);
    Lgrayi=medfilt2(Lgrayi,[3 3]);
    Lgrayi=IMCROP(Lgrayi,RECT);
    LPSNR(i,2)=20*log10(1)-10*log10( sum(sum(
(mean(Lgrayi(:)) - Lgrayi).^2 )) ./ (size(Lgrayi,1) *
size(Lgrayi,2)) );

    Lgrayi=mat2gray(L1.L1);
    Lgrayi=medfilt2(Lgrayi,[5 5]);
    Lgrayi=IMCROP(Lgrayi,RECT);
    LPSNR(i,3)=20*log10(1)-10*log10( sum(sum(
(mean(Lgrayi(:)) - Lgrayi).^2 )) ./ (size(Lgrayi,1) *
size(Lgrayi,2)) );
    Lgrayi=mat2gray(L1.L1);
    Lgrayi=medfilt2(Lgrayi,[9 9]);
    Lgrayi=IMCROP(Lgrayi,RECT);
    LPSNR(i,4)=20*log10(1)-10*log10( sum(sum(
(mean(Lgrayi(:)) - Lgrayi).^2 )) ./ (size(Lgrayi,1) *
size(Lgrayi,2)) );
    Lgrayi=mat2gray(L1.L1);
    Lgrayi=medfilt2(Lgrayi,[11 11]);
    Lgrayi=IMCROP(Lgrayi,RECT);
    LPSNR(i,5)=20*log10(1)-10*log10( sum(sum(
(mean(Lgrayi(:)) - Lgrayi).^2 )) ./ (size(Lgrayi,1) *
size(Lgrayi,2)) );
    waitbar(i/128)
end
```

```
close(hObj)
figure
plot(LPSNR(:,1),'-r*'); grid on; hold on
plot(LPSNR(:,2),'-g*');
plot(LPSNR(:,3),'-b*');
plot(LPSNR(:,4),'-m*');
plot(LPSNR(:,5),'-k*');
xlabel('i [pixel]','FontSize',14,'FontAngle','Italic')
ylabel('L_{PSNR}
[dB]','FontSize',14,'FontAngle','Italic')
legend('None','3x3','5x5','9x9','11x11')
```

The first part of the code allows to identify the *ROI* in the image $i = 80$. Then, the images from $i = 1$ to 128 are loaded sequentially from the disk and the *ROI* is separated. Then, the value of PSNR after median filtering with different mask sizes is calculated.

The results shown in Fig. 3.2 could suggest that increasing the size of the mask h_w of the median filter to the value of $M_w \times N_w = 11 \times 11$ pixels and more is the right approach. The attentive reader probably drew attention to the formulas (3.7) and (3.8), where due to the lack of the source image (devoid of noise), the mean value of $L_{MEAN}(i)$ is taken into account. These calculations are only justified when a homogeneous *ROI* is analysed and there is no source image free from noise. In other cases, the formulas (3.7) and (3.8) must be modified by replacing $L_{MEAN}(i)$ with an image devoid of noise. Since there is no noise-free image, it will be artificially added to the existing i images in gray levels. The function imnoise enables to add Gaussian or salt and pepper noise to the image $L_{GRAY}(m, n, i)$. The resulting image $L_{NOISE}(m, n, i)$ will be further used to test changes in PSNR but for the entire image (without the need to manually select the *ROI*). Filtration efficiency is here compared with the adaptive median filter, median filter and image without filtration. The source code of the m-file GUI_hyperspectral_filter_test2 allowing for this type of calculations is shown below:

```
hObj=waitbar(0,'Please wait...');
LPSNR=[]; LSEU=[];
for i=1:128
    L1=load(['D:/k/_I20_L0-511_13-1-
2016_13.5.59.cube',mat2str(i),'.mat']);
    Lgrayi=mat2gray(L1.L1);Lgrayi_=Lgrayi;
    Lnoise=imnoise(Lgrayi,'salt & pepper',0.5);
    LPSNR(i,1)=20*log10(1)-10*log10( sum(sum( (Lnoise
- Lgrayi).^2 )) ./ (size(Lgrayi,1) * size(Lgrayi,2))
);

[Lnoise_a,LSE]=GUI_hyperspectral_adaptive_filter(Lnois
e);
    LSEU(i,1:4)=hist(LSE(:),[0 3 5 7]);

    LPSNR(i,2)=20*log10(1)-10*log10( sum(sum(
(Lnoise_a - Lgrayi).^2 )) ./ (size(Lgrayi,1) *
size(Lgrayi,2)) );

    Lnoise_m=medfilt2(Lnoise,[7 7]);
    LPSNR(i,3)=20*log10(1)-10*log10( sum(sum(
(Lnoise_m - Lgrayi).^2 )) ./ (size(Lgrayi,1) *
size(Lgrayi,2)) );
    if i==80
        figure; imshow([Lgrayi,Lnoise,Lnoise_a]);
        figure; imshow([Lgrayi,Lnoise,Lnoise_m]);
    end
    waitbar(i/128)
end
close(hObj)
figure
plot(LPSNR(:,1),'-r*'); grid on; hold on
plot(LPSNR(:,2),'-g*');
plot(LPSNR(:,3),'-b*');
xlabel('i [pixel]','FontSize',14,'FontAngle','Italic')
ylabel('L_{PSNR}
[dB]','FontSize',14,'FontAngle','Italic')
legend('None','Adaptive','Median 3x3')
LSEU=LSEU./(size(Lgrayi,1) * size(Lgrayi,2))*100;
figure
plot(LSEU(:,2),'-r*'); grid on; hold on
plot(LSEU(:,3),'-g*');
plot(LSEU(:,4),'-b*');
xlabel('i [pixel]','FontSize',14,'FontAngle','Italic')
ylabel('L_{SEU}(i)
[%]','FontSize',14,'FontAngle','Italic')
legend('3x3','5x5','7x7')
```

The function GUI_hyperspectral_adaptive_filter is implemented with adaptive median filtering with a mask h_w whose size ranges from $M_w \times N_w = 3 \times 3$ pixels to $M_w \times N_w = 7 \times 7$ pixels. The main idea of the proposed adaptive filtering is to calculate erosion (image $L_{GRAYE}(m, n, i)$), dilation (image $L_{GRAYD}(m, n, i)$) and perform median filtering (image $L_{MED}(m, n, i)$) with a structural element SE_w (in the case of erosion and dilation) and a mask h_w (in the case of filtration) sized 3×3, 5×5 and 7×7 pixels, i.e.:

$$L_{GRAYE}(m,n,i) = \min_{m_{SEw},n_{SEw} \in SEw} \left(L_{GRAY}(m + m_{SEw}, n + n_{SEw}, i) \right) \qquad (3.9)$$

$$L_{GRAYD}(m,n,i) = \max_{m_{SEw},n_{SEw} \in SEw} \left(L_{GRAY}(m + m_{SEw}, n + n_{SEw}, i) \right) \qquad (3.10)$$

In order to calculate the resulting image $L_{MED}^{(c)}(m, n, i)$ after filtration with the adaptive median filter, auxiliary variables (binary images) $L_{cw}(m, n, i)$, $L_{gw}(m, n, i)$ and the image in gray levels $L_{ow}(m, n, i)$ need to be introduced:

$$L_{cw}(m,n,i) = \begin{cases} 1 & if & \left(L_{GRAYE}(m,n,i) < L_{MED}(m,n,i) \right) \wedge \\ & & \left(L_{GRAYD}(m,n,i) > L_{MED}(m,n,i) \right) \\ 0 & other \end{cases} \qquad (3.11)$$

$$L_{gw}(m,n,i) = \begin{cases} 1 & if & \left(L_{GRAYE}(m,n,i) < L_{GRAY}(m,n,i) \right) \\ & & \wedge \left(L_{GRAYD}(m,n,i) > L_{GRAY}(m,n,i) \right) \\ 0 & other \end{cases} \qquad (3.12)$$

$$L_{ow}(m,n,i) = \begin{cases} L_{MED}(m,n,i) & if & \left(L_{cw}(m,n,i) = 1 \right) \wedge \left(L_{gw}(m,n,i) = 0 \right) \\ 0 & other \end{cases}$$

$$(3.13)$$

where $L_{MED}(m, n, i)$ is the result of filtration of the image $L_{GRAY}(m, n, i)$ for the mask sized $M_w \times N_w$. In order to simplify the notation of the results of filtration, erosion and dilation carried out for a specific mask size, the size $M_w = N_w$ was given as one number as a subscript, for example, $L_{MED,3}(m, n, i)$ is the result of median filtering with a mask sized $M_w \times N_w = 3 \times 3$ pixels. Thus, the resulting image $L_{MED}^{(c)}(m, n, i)$ is equal to:

$$L_{MED}^{(c)}(m,n,i) = \begin{cases} L_{ow,5}(m,n,i) & if & \left(L_{cw,3}(m,n,i) = 0 \right) \wedge \left(L_{cw,5}(m,n,i) = 1 \right) \\ L_{ow,7}(m,n,i) & if & \left(L_{cw,3}(m,n,i) = 0 \right) \wedge \left(L_{cw,5}(m,n,i) = 0 \right) \\ L_{ow,3}(m,n,i) & other \end{cases}$$

$$(3.14)$$

The individual subscripts, e.g. 3, (as mentioned above) are directly related to the size of the mask (structural element) amounting to, for example, 3 × 3 pixels. Adaptive filtration is performed by the afore-mentioned and already used function GUI_hyperspectral_adaptive_filter with the following source code:

```
function
[Lout,LSE]=GUI_hyperspectral_adaptive_filter(Lgrayi)
Lout3=Lgrayi;
Lout5=Lgrayi;
Lout7=Lgrayi;
LSE=zeros(size(Lgrayi));
SE3=ones(3);
SE5=ones(5);
SE7=ones(7);
Lgrayei3=imerode(Lgrayi,SE3);
Lgrayei5=imerode(Lgrayi,SE5);
Lgrayei7=imerode(Lgrayi,SE7);
Lgraydi3=imdilate(Lgrayi,SE3);
Lgraydi5=imdilate(Lgrayi,SE5);
Lgraydi7=imdilate(Lgrayi,SE7);
Lmedi3=medfilt2(Lgrayi,size(SE3));
Lmedi5=medfilt2(Lgrayi,size(SE5));
Lmedi7=medfilt2(Lgrayi,size(SE7));
Lc3=(Lgrayei3<Lmedi3) & (Lgraydi3>Lmedi3);
Lc5=(Lgrayei5<Lmedi5) & (Lgraydi3>Lmedi5);
Lc7=(Lgrayei7<Lmedi7) & (Lgraydi3>Lmedi7);
Lg3=(Lgrayei3<Lgrayi) & (Lgraydi3>Lgrayi);
Lg5=(Lgrayei5<Lgrayi) & (Lgraydi5>Lgrayi);
Lg7=(Lgrayei7<Lgrayi) & (Lgraydi7>Lgrayi);
Lout3( (Lc3==1) & (Lg3==0) )=Lmedi3( (Lc3==1) &
(Lg3==0) );
Lout5( (Lc5==1) & (Lg5==0) )=Lmedi5( (Lc5==1) &
(Lg5==0) );
Lout7( (Lc7==1) & (Lg7==0) )=Lmedi7( (Lc7==1) &
(Lg7==0) );
Lout=Lout3;
Lout((Lc3==0)&(Lc5==1))=Lout5((Lc3==0)&(Lc5==1));
Lout((Lc3==0)&(Lc5==0))=Lout7((Lc3==0)&(Lc5==0));
LSE((Lc3==1) & (Lg3==0))=3;
LSE((Lc3==0)&(Lc5==1))=5;
LSE((Lc3==0)&(Lc5==0))=7;
```

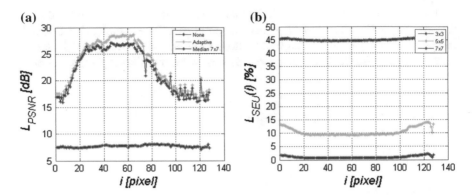

Fig. 3.3 Results of analysis of $L_{PSNR}(i)$ and $L_{SEU}(i)$ for all i images $L_{GRAY}(m,n,i)$. The graph **a** shows the measurement results of $L_{PSNR}(i)$ without filtration, with adaptive filtration and with median filtration. The graph **b** shows the values of $L_{SEU}(i)$, the percentage share in filtration of the masks sized $M_w \times N_w = 3 \times 3, 5 \times 5, 7 \times 7$ pixels

The above source code has a block structure associated with conducting triple calculations of individual variables for three different mask sizes, i.e.: $3 \times 3, 5 \times 5,$ 7×7 pixels. These calculations are necessary to determine the final form of the image $L_{MED}^{(c)}(m, n, i)$ in accordance with the formula (3.14). This function, with the source code mentioned above, provides practically relevant results—Fig. 3.3.

The results of analysis of $L_{PSNR}(i)$ values presented in Fig. 3.3(a) clearly indicate the advantage of applying an adaptive median filter over the conventional median filter with a mask sized 7×7 pixels (a difference of about 3 dB for $i \in (40,60)$) and compared to an image without any interference (filtration). Figure 3.3 b) shows the percentage share with respect to all pixels in the image $L_{GRAY}(m, n, i)$ of individual masks $M_w \times N_w = 3 \times 3, 5 \times 5, 7 \times 7$ pixels. As can be seen in Fig. 3.3(b), the share of the mask sized 3×3 pixels is the largest, about 45%. Additionally, the percentage share of the mask sized 5×5 pixels is similar to the distribution shown in Fig. 3.2. For extreme images (extreme values of i), more filtration is required, while the middle ones require less filtration. In each case of filtration, sample images and their visual assessment are much more convincing than PSNR. Therefore, Fig. 3.4 shows the images $L_{NOISE}(m, n, i)$ and $L_{MED,7}(m, n, i)$ as well as $L_{MED}^{(c)}(m, n, i)$.

The problem presented at the beginning of this subchapter, i.e.: adaptation of the filter size to the 2D image content independently for each i-th image and adaptation to the i-th 2D image depending on the wavelength, is solved by the above adaptive approach. Therefore, there is no need to develop two separate algorithms.

The presented adaptive filtration was not deliberately included in the GUI or the *m-files* of the program. At this point, I encourage the reader to make the appropriate changes in the files GUI_hyperspectral and GUI_hyperspectral_fun so that adaptive filtering will be available in the main application menu.

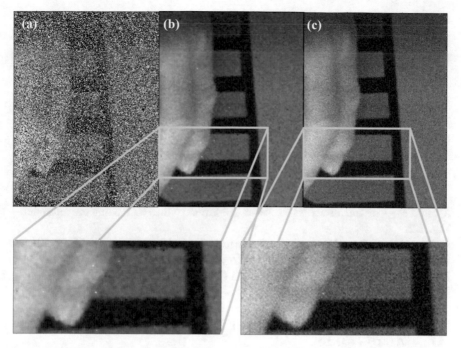

Fig. 3.4 Results of analysis for a sample image $i = 80$ **a** input image $L_{GRAY}(m, n, i = 80)$; **b** result of median filtering $L_{MED}(m, n, i = 80)$ for the mask sized $M_w \times N_w = 7 \times 7$ pixels; **c** result of adaptive median filtering $L_{MED}^{(c)}(m, n, i = 80)$

3.3 Image Calibration

Calibration of hyperspectral images is a very important element, because it is affected by many factors that can introduce significant errors to the interpretation of results (the read intensity). In practice, assuming constant light intensity in the full spectral range of the camera, there are two methods of calibration:

- using a reference visible in the analysed image or
- using calibrating images.

In the first case, calibration is related to image normalization from the value of minimum brightness occurring in the image to the mean value read from the area visible in the reference image. Therefore, the file after calibration $L_{CAL}(m,n,i)$ is calculated as:

$$L_{CAL}(m, n, i) = \frac{L_{CA2}(m, n, i)}{\max\limits_{n}\left(\max\limits_{m} L_{CA2}(m, n, i)\right)} \tag{3.15}$$

where:

$$L_{CA2}(m,n,i) = \begin{cases} L_{GRAY}(m,n,i) & if & L_{GRAY}(m,n,i) < Cal_w(i) \\ \max_n\left(\max_m L_{GRAY}(m,n,i)\right) & other \end{cases}$$

(3.16)

and:

$$Cal_w(i) = \frac{1}{M_c \cdot N_c} \sum_{m,n \in ROIc} L_{GRAY}(m,n,i)$$

(3.17)

Mc and Nc—are the numbers of rows and columns of the $ROIc$ being the reference—Fig. 2.2.

The size of the $ROIc$ is most often $Mc \times Nc = 40 \times 40$ pixels. The calibrated image $L_{CAL}(m, n, i)$ has values (for bright pixels) limited from the top by the mean brightness from the area of the reference $Cal_w(i)$. Implementation of this fragment in Matlab is simple:

```
if get(hObj(11),'Value')==1
if min(rc(2:3))>1

Cal_w=mean(mean(L1(rc(2):(rc(2)+rc(4)),rc(1):(rc(1)+rc
(3))))));
    L1(L1>Cal_w)=Cal_w;
    L1=mat2gray(L1);
end
end
```

Four values stored in the variable rc come from manual selection of the $ROIc$. It must be made clear that this calibration method can be fully automated with a constant position of the reference—e.g. always in the upper left corner of the stage. In this case, it is enough to assign the variable rc to 4 constants—x and y coordinates and the size of the $ROIc$ in x- and y-axis.

In the second case, calibration is related to the performance of 2 additional registrations of images $L_{DARK}(m, n, i)$ and $L_{WHITE}(m, n, i)$. The idea of this calibration is shown in Fig. 3.5.

These images (Fig. 3.5) are the basis for calibration. The calibrated image $L_{CAL}^{(2)}(m, n, i)$ is calculated as:

$$L_{CAL}^{(2)}(m,n,i) = \frac{L_{GRAY}(m,n,i) - L_{DARK}(m,n,i)}{\max_n\left(\max_m(L_{GRAY}(m,n,i) - L_{DARK}(m,n,i))\right)} \cdot L_{WHITE}(m,n,i)$$

(3.18)

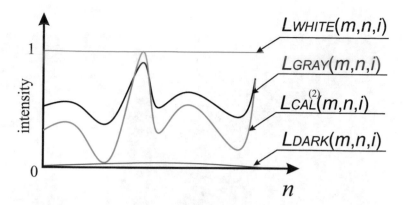

Fig. 3.5 Schematic graph of calibration results for $L_{CAL}^{(2)}(m, n, i)$ of brightness changes in the image $L_{GRAY}(m, n, i)$ using the images $L_{DARK}(m, n, i)$ and $L_{WHITE}(m, n, i)$ when $m = $ const

I encourage the reader to implement this second calibration method in practice. In this case, the reader should duplicate the reading of files in the GUI and add the relevant fragment in the file GUI_hyperspectral_fun. The further course of action and the algorithm fragment remain unchanged.

3.4   Preliminary Version of the GUI

The issues of data reading and image pre-processing presented in the previous chapters have been linked with the preparation of a preliminary version of the GUI. The GUI has been divided into several areas—Fig. 3.6.

The GUI presented in Fig. 3.6 allows for opening *.cube, *.raw or *.dat files, automatic conversion to *.mat files, reordering of image rows and columns, normalization, image rotation, artificial colouring of images, median filtering, visualization of the number of image columns and rows as well as the number of images for individual wavelengths, viewing and analysis of individual images, viewing the analysed image, displaying changes in the mean, minimum and maximum brightness for the entire area or the selected *ROI* for individual images, selecting the *ROI*, image calibration, displaying text data on the wavelength and the file name.

This GUI will be further expanded and its functionality will be increased.

3.5   Block Diagram of the Discussed Transformations

The discussed transformations along with the source code excerpts and the corresponding *m-files* can be presented in the form of a block diagram. This diagram is shown in Fig. 3.7.

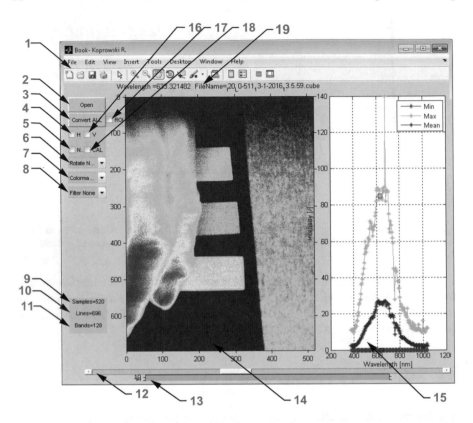

Fig. 3.6 Main menu of the application: *1* default window menu; *2* open button; *3* conversion button; *4* reordering image rows; *5* normalization; *6* image rotation; *7* artificial colour palette; *8* median filter size; *9* number of samples (number of columns); *10* number of lines (number of rows); *11* number of bands (number of images for each wavelength); *12* slider for viewing and analysis of individual images; *13* image showing the amount of converted images **.mat*; *14* viewing the analysed image; *15* graph of the mean, minimum and maximum brightness for the entire area or the selected *ROI*; *16* reordering of image columns; *17* option of selecting the *ROI*; *18* calibration; *19* text data on the wavelength and the file name

The algorithm discussed so far has been divided into three blocks: image acquisition, image pre-processing and image processing discussed later in this monograph.

The *m-files* containing the discussed functions and methods are available in this book as an attachment. It should be borne in mind that the files will be further expanded to add new functionality. For this reason, a container has been developed for readers interested in testing the discussed scope of functionality of the proposed algorithms. The container includes the discussed functions in *GUI_ver_pre.zip* attached to the book.

Fig. 3.7 Block diagram of
the initial version of the
algorithm. The block diagram
has been divided into three
main parts: image acquisition,
image pre-processing and
image processing discussed
later in this monograph. This
diagram includes one of the
blocks highlighted in blue
whose functionality has not
been deliberately included in
the main application

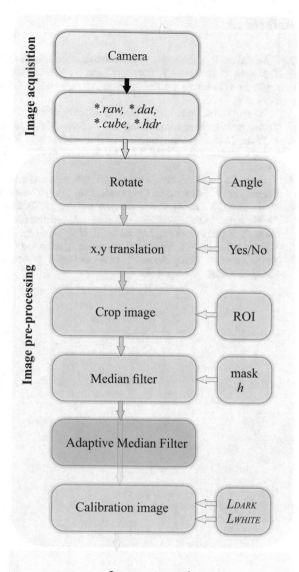

Image processing

References

1. J. Astola and P. Kuosmanen, "Fundamentals of Nonlinear Digital Filtering", CRC Press, 1997.
2. T. Sun, M. Gabbouj and Y. Neuvo, "Center weighted median filters: Some properties and their applications in image processing", Signal Processing, vol. 35, Issue 3, pp 213–229, February 1994.
3. T. Chen, K. K. Ma, L.H. Chen, "Tri-State Median Filter for Image Denoising", IEEE Transactions on Image Processing, vol. 8, Issue 12, pp 1834–1838, 1999.
4. Z. Wang, D. Zhang, "Progressive switching median filter for the removal of impulse noise from highly corrupted images", IEEE Transactions on Circuits and Systems, vol. 46, Issue 1, pp 78–80, 1999.
5. Y. Zhao, D. Li, Z. Li, "Performance enhancement and analysis of an adaptive median filter", International Conference on Communications and Networking, pp. 651–653, 2007.
6. V. Backman, R. Gurjar, K. Badizadegan, I. Itzkan, R. R. Dasari, L.T. Perelman and M.S. Feld, "A New Fast and Efficient Decision-Based Algorithm for Removal of High-Density Impulse Noises", Signal Processing Letters, IEEE, Vol. 14, Issue 3, pp 189–192, 2007.
7. V.R. Vijaykumar, P.T. Vanathi, P. Kanagasabapathy and D. Ebenezer, "High Density Impulse Noise Removal Using Robust Estimation Based Filter", IAENG International Journal of Computer Science, August 2008.

Chapter 4
Image Processing

4.1 Diagnostic Expectations

One of the key elements in the construction of the image processing algorithm is the diagnostic usefulness of the results. The literature review presented in the introduction and the publications from [1–4] show that there is a wide range of segmentation methods. Due to the large amount of information extracted from hyperspectral images, there are virtually no restrictions (relating to the minimum amount of data) to use any method of image analysis and segmentation. Therefore, many authors use segmentation methods (also used in classification) such as support vector machines (SVM) [1, 2], the nearest neighbours [3] and others [4]. These segmentation methods are based primarily on a set of data obtained from the manually selected for all acquired wavelengths. From a practical, dermatological, point of view, these methods used in hyperspectral imaging should:

- allow for segmentation of objects,
- allow for spectral analysis of any image portion,
- enable to compare the spectral characteristics of any two areas,
- allow for building a classifier based on binary decision trees, discriminant analysis and others,
- test the created classifier for different images.

© Springer International Publishing AG 2017
R. Koprowski, *Processing of Hyperspectral Medical Images*,
Studies in Computational Intelligence 682,
DOI 10.1007/978-3-319-50490-2_4

In addition, the methods used in dermatology and biomedical engineering in the field of hyperspectral imaging should be fully automatic, provide reproducible results, allow for batch data analysis (selecting only a catalogue), and be resistant to individual variability of patients. Given these expectations, both diagnostic and functional, image processing presented in the following sections has been proposed.

4.2   Tracking Changes in the Shape of an Object

An extremely important element in hyperspectral imaging is the analysis of the object/objects. This analysis is determined by the method of selecting the object. Besides simple selection of the *ROI*, automatic selection is often used in practice. Automatic selection is simply binarization or another more advanced method of segmentation. However, regardless of the segmentation method, a hyperspectral image sequence, by definition, does not provide the same image for different wavelengths. Accordingly, the segmentation process typically occurs for one of the images and its result (binary image) is used for the subsequent images. The object shape hardly ever remains the same in successive images. Therefore the only solution is to perform 3D segmentation. However, this type of segmentation requires the analysis of the entire sequence of cube images sized, for example, $M \times N \times I = 696 \times 520 \times 128$ pixels. In most types of computer programs, it is not possible due to the large amount of data for analysis (≈ 100 MB for *data type* $= 12$). Therefore, one possible solution to such problems is to track changes in the shape of an object for the successive images. One possibility is to use the methods of conditional erosion and dilation. These methods are typically used to improve the quality of binary images obtained (most often) by binarization.

Tracking changes in the shape of an object requires:

- indicating the image that will be the basis for segmentation (binarization),
- indicating the algorithm enabling the correction of the object in the binarized image relative to the other images in gray levels, for subsequent wavelengths.

The method of conditional erosion and dilation involves designation of one of the images $L_{GRAY}(m, n, i)$, most often for $i = 1$, and then segmentation, for example, using binarization with a threshold p_{bg}, providing the image $L_{BIN}(m, n, i)$, i.e.:

$$L_{BIN}(m, n, i) = \begin{cases} 1 & if \quad L_{GRAY}(m, n, i) > p_{bg} \\ 0 & other \end{cases} \qquad (4.1)$$

As a consequence, two images are obtained (e.g. for $i = 1$), namely $L_{GRAY}(m, n, i = 1)$ and $L_{BIN}(m, n, i = 1)$. Let us assume that there is only one object in the binary image $L_{BIN}(m, n, i = 1)$. Conditional erosion and dilation for the adopted symmetric structural element $SE2(m_{SE2}, n_{SE2})$ sized $M_{SE2} \times N_{SE2}$ are shown below:

$$L_{BINE}^{(C)}(m, n, i)$$
$$= \begin{cases} L_{BIN}(m, n, 1) & if \quad p_c(m, n, i) < p_{dc} \quad (4.2) \\ \min_{m_{SE2}, n_{SE2} \in SE2} (L_{BIN}(m + m_{SE2}, n + n_{SE2}, i)) & other \end{cases}$$

$$L_{BIND}^{(C)}(m, n, i) = \begin{cases} L_{BIN}^{(m,n,1)} & if \quad p_c(m, n, i) > p_{ec} \\ \max_{m_{SE2}, n_{SE2} \in SE2} (L_{BIN}(m + m_{SE2}, n + n_{SE2}, i)) & other \end{cases}$$

$$(4.3)$$

where

$$p_c(m, n, i) = \frac{1}{M_{SE2} \cdot N_{SE2}} \sum_{m_{SE2}=1}^{M_{SE2}} \sum_{n_{SE2}=1}^{N_{SE2}} L_{GRAY}(m + m_{SE2}, n + n_{SE2}, i) \quad (4.4)$$

as well as p_{ec} and p_{dc}—the thresholds set by the user.

The constants p_{ec} and p_{dc} determining the effectiveness of erosion and dilation respectively take values dependent on the type of the variable in which the image $L_{GRAY}(m, n, i)$ is stored. In the case of the variable type double, these are values from the range $p_e = p_d \in (0, 1)$, whereas for the variable type uint8—$p_e = p_d$ (0, 255). The corresponding source codes for erosion and dilation are shown below —these are functions GUI_hyperspectral_dilate_c and GUI_hyperspectral_erode_c:

```
function
[Lbind]=GUI_hyperspectral_dilate_c(Lgray,Lbin,se2,pdc,
vi)
...
[sm,sn]=size(se2);
[m,n]=size(Lbin);
ppp=floor(([sm,sn]+1)/2); pm=ppp(1); pn=ppp(2);
if vi==1
    hg = waitbar(0,'Working.... ');
end
Lbind=Lbin;
for mm=1:(m-sm)
    for nn=1:(n-sn)
        Lsu=sum(sum(Lbin(  mm : (mm+sm-1) , nn :
(nn+sn-1)  ).*se2  ));
        if Lsu<sum(se2(:))
        if Lsu>0
        if Lbin(mm+pm-1,nn+pn-1)==1;
            wyy=Lgray(  mm : (mm+sm-1) , nn : (nn+sn-1)
);
            if sum(sum(  wyy .*se2
))/sum(sum(se2>0)))>pdc;
                Lbind(  mm : (mm+sm-1) , nn : (nn+sn-1)
)=se2;
            end
        end
        end
        end
    end
if vi==1
    waitbar(mm/(m-sm),hg)
end
end
if vi==1
    close(hg)
end
```

Analogously for dilation, i.e.:

```
function
[Lbine]=GUI_hyperspectral_erode_c(Lgray,Lbin,se2,pec,v
i)
...
[sm,sn]=size(se2);
[m,n]=size(Lbin);
if vi==1
    hg = waitbar(0,'Working....');
end
Lbine=Lbin;
for mm=1:(m-sm)
    for nn=1:(n-sn)
        Lsu=sum(sum(Lbin(  mm : (mm+sm-1) , nn :
(nn+sn-1)  ).*se2  ));
        if Lsu<sum(se2(:))
        if Lsu>0
        if Lbin( round((mm+sm-1+mm)/2) , round((nn+sn-
1+nn)/2) )==1;
            wyy=Lgray(  mm : (mm+sm-1) , nn : (nn+sn-1)
);
            if sum(sum(  wyy .*se2
))/sum(sum(se2>0))<pec;
                Lbine(  mm : (mm+sm-1) , nn : (nn+sn-1)
)=0;
            end
        end
        end
        end
    end
if vi==1
    waitbar(mm/(m-sm),hg)
end
end
if vi==1
    close(hg);
end
```

The described functions of conditional opening and closing do not fulfil, in comparison with the classical approach, the following relationships:

• subsequent operations of opening or closing may cause further changes in the size of the object in the image, i.e.:

$$(L_{BIN}(m,n,i) \ominus SE2) \oplus SE2$$
$$\neq (((L_{BIN}(m,n,i) \ominus SE2) \oplus SE2) \ominus SE2) \oplus SE2 \qquad (4.5)$$

$$(L_{BIN}(m,n,i) \oplus SE2) \ominus SE2$$
$$\neq (((L_{BIN}(m,n,i) \oplus SE2) \ominus SE2) \oplus SE2) \ominus SE2 \qquad (4.6)$$

where symbols $\ominus, \oplus$ refer to erosion and dilation respectively.

- opening the image completeness is not equal to the completeness of its closing and vice versa, i.e.:

$$\left(L_{BIN}^{(D)}(m,n,i) \ominus SE2\right) \oplus SE2 \neq \left(\left(L_{BIN}^{(D)}(m,n,i) \oplus SE2\right) \ominus SE2\right)^{(D)} \qquad (4.7)$$

$$\left(\left(L_{BIN}^{(D)}(m,n,i) \ominus SE2\right) \oplus SE2\right)^{(D)} \neq \left(L_{BIN}^{(D)}(m,n,i) \oplus SE2\right) \ominus SE2 \qquad (4.8)$$

where

$L_{BIN}^{(D)}$—completeness (superscript D) of the image L_{BIN},

- the images resulting from opening for the included structural elements 'a' and 'b' do not need to be included, i.e.:

$$\left(L_{BIN}^{(a)}(m,n,i) \ominus SE2\right) \oplus SE2 \not\subset \left(L_{BIN}^{(b)}(m,n,i) \ominus SE2\right) \oplus SE2 \qquad (4.9)$$

$$\left(L_{BIN}^{(a)}(m,n,i) \oplus SE2\right) \ominus SE2 \not\subset \left(L_{BIN}^{(b)}(m,n,i) \oplus SE2\right) \ominus SE2 \qquad (4.10)$$

where $L_{BIN}^{(a)} \subseteq L_{BIN}^{(b)}$.

Specificity of the described conditional erosion and dilation operations is based on the sequential performance of conditional erosion and dilation, i.e.:

$$L_{BIN}^{(F)}(m,n,i)$$
$$= (((((L_{BIN}(m,n,i) \ominus SE2) \oplus SE2) \ominus SE2) \oplus SE2) \ominus SE2 \qquad (4.11)$$

The number of performed sequential operations of conditional erosion and dilation strictly depends on the size of the structural element $SE2$ and the shape of the object in the binary image $L_{BIN}(m,n,i)$. Figure 4.1 shows changes in the surface area for successive iterations and various values of the threshold $p_{ec} = p_{dc}$

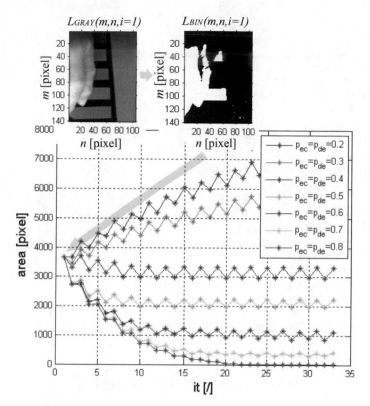

Fig. 4.1 Changes in the surface area for successive iterations and various values of the threshold $p_{ec} = p_{dc}$

$\in$ {0.2, 0.3, ..., 0.7, 0.8} for a sample object with the total surface area of 3667 pixels. It also shows the first images $L_{GRAY}(m, n, i = 1)$ and $L_{BIN}(m, n, i = 1)$ for which the calculations were made.

Figure 4.1 shows three different situations. The first one is the complete removal of the object from the image obtained for $p_{ec} = p_{dc} = 0.8$. The second one is the adjustment of the position and shape of the object visible when $p_{ec} = p_{dc} \in$ {0.4, 0.5, 0.6, 0.7}. The third one is zooming the object to the full size of the image for $p_{ec} = p_{dc} \in$ {0.2, 0.3}. The source code providing the above graph is shown below:

```
L1=load('D:/k/_I20_L0-511_13-1-
2016_13.5.59.cube50.mat');
Lgray=mat2gray(L1.L1);
Lgray=imresize(Lgray,0.2);
Lbin=Lgray>0.4;
figure; imshow(Lbin)

L1=load('D:/k/_I20_L0-511_13-1-
2016_13.5.59.cube80.mat');
Lgray=mat2gray(L1.L1);
Lgray=imresize(Lgray,0.2);
figure; imshow(Lgray,[])

Lorg=Lbin;
se2=ones(3); pam=[];
for pec=0.2:0.1:0.8;
    vi=1; Lbin=Lorg;
    pami=[];
    pami=[pami;[0, sum(sum(Lbin))]];
    for it=1:16

[Lbin]=GUI_hyperspectral_erode_c(Lgray,Lbin,se2,pec,vi
);
%          imshow(Lbin)
%          pause(0.1)
        pami=[pami;[it, sum(sum(Lbin))]];

[Lbin]=GUI_hyperspectral_dilate_c(Lgray,Lbin,se2,pec,v
i);
%          imshow(Lbin)
%          pause(0.1)
        pami=[pami;[it, sum(sum(Lbin))]];
    end
    pam=[pam,pami(:,2)];
end
figure; plot(pam,'-*'); grid on
xlabel('it [/]','FontSize',14)
ylabel('area [pixel]','FontSize',14)
leg-
end('p_{ec}=p_{de}=0.2','p_{ec}=p_{de}=0.3','p_{ec}=p_
{de}=0.4','p_{ec}=p_{de}=0.5','p_{ec}=p_{de}=0.6','p_{
ec}=p_{de}=0.7','p_{ec}=p_{de}=0.8')
```

In the above source code, a change in the value of p_{ec} and p_{dc} ranging from 0.2 to 0.8 in each loop circulation is noteworthy. Then, according to the idea presented above, conditional erosion and dilation, functions GUI_hyper-spectral_dilate_c and GUI_hyperspectral_erode_c, are calculated alternately.

The assessment of the convergence of the algorithm should be carried out also for other sizes of the structural element *SE2* (in the present case it was 3×3 pixels). A more detailed analysis of the various types of collected images and various sizes of objects confirmed that typically the convergence of the algorithm can be reached after approximately 15 iterations, when fluctuations around the correct value of the surface area are in the range of $\pm 10\%$ (quasi steady state). An increase in the size of the structural element *SE2* increases the rate of convergence but also the error of approximately $\pm 40\%$ in relation to the object separated by an expert. The accuracy of 10% is usually obtained if the size of the structural element *SE2* constitutes $\cong 3\%$ of the object surface area. This relationship is clearly visible in Fig. 4.2a which shows a graph of changes in the surface area of the object for subsequent iterations and resizing the structural element *SE2* from 3×3 pixels to 11×11 pixels.

The other graphs in Fig. 4.2b–d show the results for the input image resolution $M \times N = 279 \times 208$ pixels, $M \times N = 557 \times 416$ pixels as well as 32 and 64

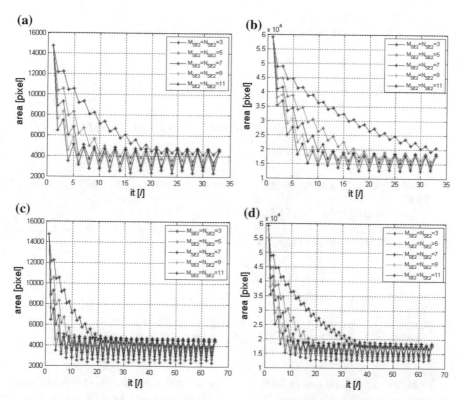

Fig. 4.2 Graph of changes in the surface area of the object for subsequent iterations and resizing the structural element *SE2* from 3×3 pixels to 11×11 pixels: **a** for $M \times N = 279 \times 208$ pixels and 32 iterations; **b** for $M \times N = 557 \times 416$ pixels and 32 iterations; **c** for $M \times N = 279 \times 208$ pixels and 64 iterations; **d** for $M \times N = 557 \times 416$ pixels and 64 iterations

iterations. The source code allowing for the calculations for the first graph presented in Fig. 4.2a is shown below:

```
L1=load('D:/k/_I20_L0-511_13-1-
2016_13.5.59.cube50.mat');
Lgray=mat2gray(L1.L1);
Lgray=imresize(Lgray,0.4);
Lbin=Lgray>0.4;
figure; imshow(Lbin)

L1=load('D:/k/_I20_L0-511_13-1-
2016_13.5.59.cube80.mat');
Lgray=mat2gray(L1.L1);
Lgray=imresize(Lgray,0.4);
figure; imshow(Lgray,[])

Lorg=Lbin;
pam=[];
for MSE2NSE2=3:2:11
    SE2=ones(MSE2NSE2);
    pec=0.6;
    vi=1; Lbin=Lorg;
    pami=[];
    pami=[pami;[0, sum(sum(Lbin))]];
    for it=1:16

[Lbin]=GUI_hyperspectral_erode_c(Lgray,Lbin,SE2,pec,vi
);
        pami=[pami;[it, sum(sum(Lbin))]];

[Lbin]=GUI_hyperspectral_dilate_c(Lgray,Lbin,SE2,pec,v
i);
        pami=[pami;[it, sum(sum(Lbin))]];
    end
    pam=[pam,pami(:,2)];
end
figure; plot(pam,'-*'); grid on
xlabel('it [/]','FontSize',14)
ylabel('area [pixel]','FontSize',14)
leg-
end('M_{SE2}=N_{SE2}=3','M_{SE2}=N_{SE2}=5','M_{SE2}=N
_{SE2}=7','M_{SE2}=N_{SE2}=9','M_{SE2}=N_{SE2}=11')
```

To better understand and illustrate the transformations in the above source code, the parts responsible for reading the image (for $i = 50$ and $i = 80$) are separated. The presented loop enables to resize the mask SE2 = ones(MSE2NSE2) in the range from 3 to 11 every 2 pixels.

For zero iteration ($it = 0$), which is the initial state, the total surface area shown in Fig. 4.2 is greater than the surface area for the same iteration shown in Fig. 4.1. This is due to the adopted change in the resolution of the input image. In the first case, the resolution is reduced to 20% of the original size, while in the second case it is 40% of the original image resolution.

Due to the nature of conditional erosion and dilation, two-dimensional image convolution, the time necessary to obtain the results depends on the image resolution, the size and shape of the object and the size of the structural element $SE2$. Some selected times of analysis are shown in Table 4.1. IT indicates the maximum number of iterations, and it^* the number of iterations after which the quasi steady state is achieved.

The time of analysis shown in Table 4.1 is affected to the greatest extent by the image resolution. According to the intuition, doubling the image resolution results in an almost fourfold increase in computation time. The structural element $SE2$ influences the calculation time to the least extent.

The results of the proposed algorithm for tracking the object based on conditional erosion and dilation are presented in Figs. 4.3 and 4.4.

Table 4.1 Some selected times of analysis for two different sizes of the object, five different sizes of the structural element and different numbers of iterations (for Intel® Xenon® CPU X5680@3.33 GHz)

Time (s)	$M \times N$ (pixel)	$M_{SE2} \times N_{SE2}$ (pixel)	IT [/]	it^* [/]
7.7	279 × 208	3 × 3	16.2	21
7.5	279 × 208	5 × 5	16.2	11
7.7	279 × 208	7 × 7	16.2	7
7.9	279 × 208	9 × 9	16.2	6
8.4	279 × 208	11 × 11	16.2	6
30.1	557 × 416	3 × 3	16.2	32
30.4	557 × 416	5 × 5	16.2	20
31.6	557 × 416	7 × 7	16.2	13
32.6	557 × 416	9 × 9	16.2	12
34	557 × 416	11 × 11	16.2	8
15.5	279 × 208	3 × 3	32.2	28
15.1	279 × 208	5 × 5	32.2	18
15.6	279 × 208	7 × 7	32.2	11
16.0	279 × 208	9 × 9	32.2	9
16.7	279 × 208	11 × 11	32.2	7
59.7	557 × 416	3 × 3	32.2	40
60.9	557 × 416	5 × 5	32.2	19
62.9	557 × 416	7 × 7	32.2	13
65.4	557 × 416	9 × 9	32.2	11
69.6	557 × 416	11 × 11	32.2	8

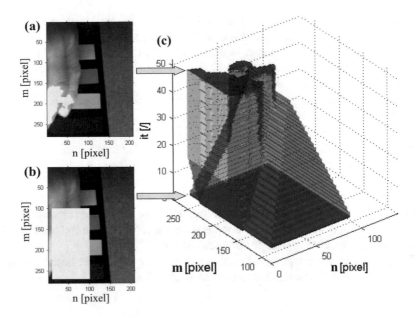

Fig. 4.3 Results of conditional erosion and dilation for an artificial binary image representing a rectangle. Part **a** shows the output image $L_{BINE}(m, n, i)$ as a binary image superimposed on the image in gray levels $L_{GRAY}(m, n, i)$. Part **b** shows the input image $L_{BINE}(m, n, i)$ as a binary image superimposed on the input image in gray levels $L_{GRAY}(m, n, i)$. Subsequent stages of erosion and dilation are shown in part (**c**) for $p_{ec} = p_{dc} = 0.8$

The results of conditional erosion and dilation presented in Figs. 4.3 and 4.4 were obtained for an artificial binary image representing a rectangle. Part a shows the output image as a binary image superimposed on the image in gray levels. Figures 4.3b and 4.4 show the input image as a binary image superimposed on the input image in gray levels. The subsequent stages of erosion and dilation are shown in Figs. 4.3c and 4.4c. These are the successive stages of conditional erosion and dilation for successive conditional erosions and dilations of the images $L_{BINE}(m, n, i)$ and $L_{BIND}(m, n, i)$. Figure 4.3 shows the results for $p_{ec} = p_{dc} = 0.8$ and Fig. 4.4 for $p_{ec} = p_{dc} = 0.4$. In both cases the size of the structural element $SE2$ was the same, namely 3×3 pixels. Therefore, Figs. 4.3 and 4.4 show how conditional erosion and dilation, which enable to change the shape of the object present in the image from a rectangle to the shape corresponding to the content of the image $L_{GRAY}(m, n, i)$, work in practice.

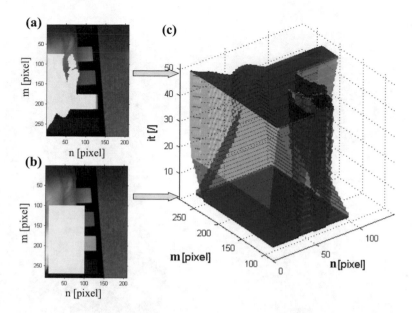

Fig. 4.4 Results of conditional erosion and dilation for an artificial binary image representing a rectangle. Part **a** shows the output image $L_{BINE}(m, n, i)$ as a binary image superimposed on the image in gray levels $L_{GRAY}(m, n, i)$. Part **b** shows the input image $L_{BINE}(m, n, i)$ as a binary image superimposed on the input image in gray levels $L_{GRAY}(m, n, i)$. Subsequent stages of erosion and dilation are shown in part (**c**) for $p_{ec} = p_{dc} = 0.4$

In this way, the above algorithm was implemented to track an object whose shape changes for successive i images in a series. To this end, setting the threshold manually or automatically, the first image $L_{GRAY}(m, n, i = 1)$ can be subjected to binarization providing the image $L_{BIN}(m, n, i = 1)$ and then, conditional erosion and dilation of the images $L_{BINE}(m, n, i \neq 1)$ and $L_{BIND}(m, n, i \neq 1)$ can be performed alternately. In practice, however, the first image ($i = 1$) is rarely used as a basis for binarization and then determination of the starting object whose shape is further corrected. This is due to the large amount of noise in the image. The middle image in a series is most commonly adopted as the value i, i.e.: $i = I/2 = 64$ (assuming an even number of I). The results are shown in Fig. 4.5.

The results of conditional erosion and dilation shown in Fig. 4.5 were obtained for successive images in a sequence for $i \in (1, I)$ and $IT = 11$. The analysis was started from the binary image $L_{BIN}(m, n, i = I/2)$. The next images in Fig. 4.5a–d

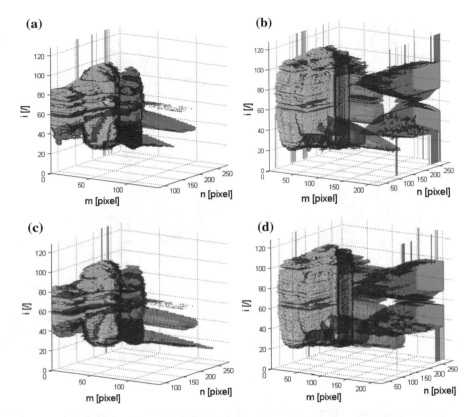

Fig. 4.5 Results of conditional erosion and dilation performed for subsequent images in a sequence for $i \in (1, I)$ and $IT = 11$ starting with the binary image $L_{BIN}(m, n, i = I/2)$ when: **a** $p_{ec} = p_{dc} = 0.5$ and $M_{SE2} \times N_{SE2} = 3 \times 3$; **b** $p_{ec} = p_{dc} = 0.3$ and $M_{SE2} \times N_{SE2} = 3 \times 3$; **c** $p_{ec} = p_{dc} = 0.5$ and $M_{SE2} \times N_{SE2} = 5 \times 5$; **d** $p_{ec} = p_{dc} = 0.3$ and $M_{SE2} \times N_{SE2} = 5 \times 5$

were obtained for $p_{ec} = p_{dc} \in \{0.3, 0.5\}$ and $M_{SE2} \times N_{SE2} \in \{3 \times 3, 5 \times 5\}$. Depending on the selected parameters of the algorithm, the shape of the tracked object changes significantly. These changes are due to the different amount of noise in the image, the individual changes in the size of the object for the adjacent 2D images etc. In each case, these parameters (p_{ec}, p_{dc}, M_{SE2}, N_{SE2}) are selected individually.

The source code for displaying the results from Fig. 4.5a is shown below:

```
L1=load('D:/k/_I20_L0-511_13-1-
2016_13.5.59.cube64.mat');
Lgray=mat2gray(L1.L1);
Lgray=imresize(Lgray,0.4);
Lbin=Lgray>0.4;
Lbini=[];
Lbini(1:size(Lbin,1),1:size(Lbin,2),64)=Lbin;
SE2=ones(5);
pec=0.5;
vi=0;
for i=65:128
    L1=load(['D:/k/_I20_L0-511_13-1-
2016_13.5.59.cube',mat2str(i),'.mat']);
    Lgray=mat2gray(L1.L1);
    Lgray=imresize(Lgray,0.4);
    for it=1:2:10

[Lbin]=GUI_hyperspectral_erode_c(Lgray,Lbin,SE2,pec,vi
);

[Lbin]=GUI_hyperspectral_dilate_c(Lgray,Lbin,SE2,pec,v
i);
        [i it]
    end
    Lbini(1:size(Lbin,1),1:size(Lbin,2),i)=Lbin;
    if (i==80)|(i==120)
        Lbeg=Lgray; Lbeg(Lbin==1)=max(Lbeg(:));
        figure; imshow(Lbeg,[]); ti-
tle(['i=',mat2str(i)])
    end
end
Lbin=Lbini(1:size(Lbin,1),1:size(Lbin,2),64);
for i=63:-1:1
    L1=load(['D:/k/_I20_L0-511_13-1-
2016_13.5.59.cube',mat2str(i),'.mat']);
    Lgray=mat2gray(L1.L1);
    Lgray=imresize(Lgray,0.4);
    for it=1:2:10

[Lbin]=GUI_hyperspectral_erode_c(Lgray,Lbin,SE2,pec,vi
);

[Lbin]=GUI_hyperspectral_dilate_c(Lgray,Lbin,SE2,pec,v
i);
        [i it]
    end
```

```
    Lbini(1:size(Lbin,1),1:size(Lbin,2),i)=Lbin;
    if (i==10)|(i==40)
        Lbeg=Lgray; Lbeg(Lbin==1)=max(Lbeg(:));
        figure; imshow(Lbeg,[]); ti-
tle(['i=',mat2str(i)])
    end
end

figure
[x,y,z]=meshgrid( 1:size(Lbini,2) , 1:size(Lbini,1) ,
1:size(Lbini,3));
p1 = patch(isosurface(x,y,z,Lbini,0.5),'FaceColor',[0
0 1 ],'EdgeColor','none');
view(33,12);
camlight; camlight(-80,-10); lighting phong;
grid on
alpha(p1,0.3)
hold on
axis square
axis([0 220 20 290 0 128])
xlabel('m [pixel]','FontSize',14)
ylabel('n [pixel]','FontSize',14)
zlabel('i [/]','FontSize',14)
```

The above source code consists of two parts. In the first one, there is a loop designed for the analysis of images from i equal to 65 to 128. This analysis involves a sequence of conditional erosions and dilations for it = 1:2:10. The other part of the source code concerns the analysis for decreasing values of i, i.e. from 63 to 1. Thus, the 2D image for $i = 64$ is the beginning of the analysis running in both directions (decreasing and increasing i).

The presented method for tracking the shape of an object was not deliberately included in the overall GUI of the described program to encourage readers to its independent implementation. The full source code shown above is attached to this monograph in the form of the following *m-files*:

```
GUI_hyperspectral_erode_dilate_test,
GUI_hyperspectral_erode_dilate_test2,
GUI_hyperspectral_erode_dilate_test3
```
and
```
GUI_hyperspectral_erode_dilate_test4.
```

4.3 Basic Analysis of Features

The basic element of hyperspectral image analysis is a comparative analysis of features such as the mean value or contrast both of the whole image and the *ROI*. In this case, two groups of data are compared.

The first group of data is derived directly from the analysed image. This may be, as previously mentioned, the mean value of brightness $L_S(i)$ of the selected ROI_S, for example [similarly to (3.17)]:

$$L_S(i) = \frac{1}{M_S \times N_S} \sum_{m,n \in ROI_S} L_{GRAY}(m, n, i) \tag{4.12}$$

It may be also the value of minimum or maximum brightness. The first group of data can be also created as a result of texture analysis. These may be, for example, the results of analysis of gray-level co-occurrence matrix (GLCM), i.e.:

$$L_{GLCM}(u, v, i) = \sum_{n=1}^{N} \sum_{m=1}^{M} L_{GB}(m, n, i, u, v) \tag{4.13}$$

where L_{GB} can be calculated for the horizontal neighbourhood (an arrow as a superscript) $L_{GB}^{\rightarrow}$:

$$L_{GB}^{\rightarrow}(m, n, i, u, v)$$
$$= \begin{cases} 1 & if \quad (L_{GRAY}(m, n, i) = u) \wedge (L_{GRAY}(m+1, n, i) = v) \\ 0 & other \end{cases} \tag{4.14}$$

for $m \in (1, M-1)$ and $n \in (1, N)$, $u \in (1, U)$ and $v \in (1, V)$ where U and V are equal to the number of brightness levels, i.e. 2^B where B is the number of bits per pixel. The above notation concerns the comparison of the horizontal neighbourhood of pixels. For the vertical arrangement, the formula (4.14) is converted to the following relationship:

$$L_{GB}^{\downarrow}(m, n, i, u, v)$$
$$= \begin{cases} 1 & if \quad (L_{GRAY}(m, n, i) = u) \wedge (L_{GRAY}(m+1, n, i) = v) \\ 0 & other \end{cases} \tag{4.15}$$

for $m \in (1, M)$ and $n \in (1, N-1)$.

On this basis ($L_{GLCM}(u, v, i)$), the parameters such as contrast $L_{CON}(i)$, energy $L_{ENE}(i)$ or homogeneity $L_{HOM}(i)$ are calculated, i.e.:

$$L_{CON}(i) = \sum_{v=1}^{V} \sum_{u=1}^{U} (v - u)^2 L_{GLCM}(u, v, i) \tag{4.16}$$

$$L_{ENE}(i) = \sum_{v=1}^{V} \sum_{u=1}^{U} L_{GLCM}(u, v, i)^2 \tag{4.17}$$

$$L_{HOM}(i) = \sum_{v=1}^{V} \sum_{u=1}^{U} \frac{1}{1 + (v - u)^2} L_{GLCM}(u, v, i) \tag{4.18}$$

Apart from analysis of GLCM, other texture features such as the surface area of the recognized references can be also analysed. In the simplest form, this is the sum $L_{DET}(i)$ of the image $L_{WZ}(m, n, i)$ after binarization using the threshold p_{rw}:

$$L_{DET}(i) = \sum_{m=1}^{M} \sum_{n=1}^{N} L_D(m, n, i) \tag{4.19}$$

where

$$L_D(m, n, i) = \begin{cases} 1 & if \quad L_{OC}(m, n, i) > p_{rw} \\ 0 & other \end{cases} \tag{4.20}$$

$$L_{OC}(m, n, i) = L_{GRAY}(m, n, i) \\ - min \left(\min_{m,n} \left(\max_{SE} \left(\max_{SE} \left(\min_{SE} (L_{GRAY}(m, n, i)) \right) \right) \right), L_{GRAY}(m, n, i) \right) \tag{4.21}$$

SE—is a structural element whose shape corresponds to the shape of the recognized reference.

All the above new features are calculated separately for each ith wavelength and will be further used.

The other group of data is derived from another portion of the same image. It can be also acquired from another image or it may be a data vector (loaded outside).

To distinguish between these two groups of data, upper indexes were introduced —'W' for the second group of data and 'E' for the first group of data. A basic comparison involves calculating the difference between the data vectors, for example, the calculated mean value of brightness, i.e.:

$$\delta_S(i) = \frac{\left| L_S^W(i) - L_S^E(i) \right|}{\max_{i \in (1,I)} L_S^W(i)} \tag{4.22}$$

Fig. 4.6 The idea of calculating *FN*, *FP*, *TP* and *TN* for a sample graph of the variable $\delta_S(i)$: **a** a graph of the mean brightness for comparable areas and their difference $\delta_S(i)$, **b** the areas marked in *red* and *green* by the user meet or do not meet the condition of compliance; **c** the results of comparisons of the *red* and *green* areas from parts (**a**) and (**b**)

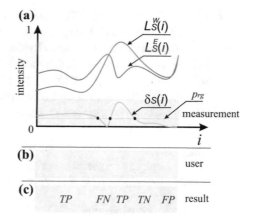

These differences are then binarized with respect to the threshold p_q that is set manually and expressed as a percentage of the value of the variable $\delta_S(i)$.

The analysis of the two discussed groups of data and the values they provide is related to the areas selected manually. On this basis, the values of *FN*, *FP*, *TP* and *TN* are calculated. The idea of these calculations is shown in Fig. 4.6.

The values of the variable $\delta_S(i)$ below the assumed threshold p_{rg} satisfy the condition of allowable differences between comparable features - in this case the mean brightness values. These wavelengths (values i) that are different or exceed the threshold p_{rg} are marked in Fig. 4.6a with a red background. Similar colours (red and green) were used to mark in Fig. 4.6b the areas that must comply with the condition of miscellaneous brightness levels below the set threshold. The following excerpt in the function GUI_hyperspectral_fun is to enable the user to manually select these areas on a graph:

```
ax=axis(hObj(21));

set(hObj(70),'XData',[ax(1)],'YData',[ax(4)],'FaceColo
r','g');

set(hObj(71),'XData',[ax(1)],'YData',[ax(4)],'FaceColo
r','r');
    re=getrect(hObj(21));
    rect=[re(1),re(1)+re(3)];
    set(hObj(70),'XData',[ax(1) rect(1) rect(1)
rect(2) rect(2) ax(2)],'YData',[ax(4) ax(4) 0 0 ax(4)
ax(4) ],'FaceColor','r');
    set(hObj(71),'XData',[rect(1)
rect(2)],'YData',[ax(4) ax(4)],'FaceColor','g');
    alpha(0.1)
```

A comparison of the two results calculated automatically and set manually is shown in Fig. 4.6c. On this basis, the aforementioned values of *FN*, *FP*, *TP* and *TN* as well as *ACC* are calculated. The usefulness of this type of analysis is very high in practical applications and diagnostics, for which the degree of compliance of the mean brightness level with the actual values is analysed.

A fragment of the source code responsible for this part of calculations is located in four *m-files* GUI_hyperspectral_diff, GUI_hyperspectral_class, GUI_hyperspectral and GUI_hyperspectral_fun. The source code of the function GUI_hyperspectral_diff is shown below:

```
function
[diff_test_reference,wavelength_reference_test]=GUI_hy
perspectral_diff(reference,test)

tw=test.Wavelength_;
td=test.anal;

pw=reference.Wavelength_;
pd=reference.anal;

twd=[tw,td];
pwd=[pw,pd];

twd(min(pwd(:,1))>twd(:,1),:)=[];
twd(max(pwd(:,1))<twd(:,1),:)=[];
pwd(min(twd(:,1))>pwd(:,1),:)=[];
pwd(max(twd(:,1))<pwd(:,1),:)=[];

if (size(twd,1)>0) && (size(pwd,1)>0)
    y1 = interp1(twd(:,1),twd(:,4),pwd(:,1));
    y2 = interp1(twd(:,1),twd(:,5),pwd(:,1));
    y3 = interp1(twd(:,1),twd(:,6),pwd(:,1));
    y4 = interp1(twd(:,1),twd(:,7),pwd(:,1));
    diff_test_reference=[twd(:,1),abs(pwd(:,4)-
y1)./max(pwd(:,4)),abs(pwd(:,5)-
y2)./max(pwd(:,5)),abs(pwd(:,6)-
y3)./max(pwd(:,6)),abs(pwd(:,7)-y4)./max(pwd(:,7))];
    wave-
length_reference_test=[twd(:,1),pwd(:,4:7),y1,y2,y3,y4
];
else
    diff_test_reference=[];
    wavelength_reference_test=[];
end
```

The presented source code can be divided into 2 elements:

- standardization of the variables test and reference so that they cover the same range of wavelengths (of the measured *i* images). This is due to the versatility of the approach for which, in any case, it is possible to perform calculations in the proposed application for any range of wavelengths.

- calculation of the values of $\delta_S(i)$ as well as $\delta_{CON}(i)$, $\delta_{ENE}(i)$ and $\delta_{HOM}(i)$ – stored in the variable diff_test_reference.

The values included in the variables test and reference are obtained using two possibilities:

- the first one is the aforementioned manual selection of the *ROI*. Manual selection of the *ROI* was realized in the fragment of the source code in the file GUI_hyperspectral_fun, i.e.:

```
if sw==14
    ax=axis(hObj(21));
set(hObj(70),'XData',[ax(1)],'YData',[ax(4)],'Fac
eColor','g');

set(hObj(71),'XData',[ax(1)],'YData',[ax(4)],'Fac
eColor','r');
    re=getrect(hObj(21));
    rect=[re(1),re(1)+re(3)];
    set(hObj(70),'XData',[ax(1) rect(1) rect(1)
rect(2) rect(2) ax(2)],'YData',[ax(4) ax(4) 0 0
ax(4) ax(4) ],'FaceColor','r');
    set(hObj(71),'XData',[rect(1)
rect(2)],'YData',[ax(4) ax(4)],'FaceColor','g');
    alpha(0.1)
    GUI_hyperspectral_fun(8)
end
```

It (the above code fragment) is invoked in the function GUI_hyperspectral in the fragment:

```
hObj(34) =uicontrol('Style', 'pushbut-
ton','units','normalized', 'String',
'SELECT','Position', [0.69 0.95 0.3 0.03],...
    'Callback',
'GUI_hyperspectral_fun(14)','BackgroundColor',col
or2);
```

- the other one is reading from the external file test.mat and/or refer- ence.mat. The code fragment of the function GUI_hyperspectral_fun is responsible for reading, i.e.:

```
if sw==6 % GET FILE TEST
        [filen_, pathn_] = uigetfile('test.mat',
'Select test.mat file');
    if isequal(filen_,0)==0
        test=load([pathn_,filen_]);
        set(hObj(35),'ForegroundColor','g')
            GUI_hyperspectral_fun(8)
    else
        set(hObj(35),'ForegroundColor','r')
        errordlg('File test.mat not found','File
Error');
    end
end
if sw==7 % GET FILE REFERENCE
        [filen_, pathn_] = uiget-
file('reference.mat', 'Select reference.mat
file');

    if isequal(filen_,0)==0
        reference=load([pathn_,filen_]);
        set(hObj(36),'ForegroundColor','g')
            GUI_hyperspectral_fun(8)
    else
        set(hObj(36),'ForegroundColor','r')
        errordlg('File reference.mat not
found','File Error');
    end
end
```

When a wrong file is indicated or no file is indicated, there appears `errordlg` saying `'File reference.mat not found'` and/or `'File test.mat not found'`. Reading is possible by placing the two buttons in the main window, in the file `GUI_hyperspectral`, i.e.:

```
hObj(37) =uicontrol('Style', 'pushbut-
ton','units','normalized', 'String',
'OPEN','Position', [0.06 0.48 0.05 0.04],...
    'Callback',
'GUI_hyperspectral_fun(6)','BackgroundColor',colo
r2);
hObj(38) =uicontrol('Style', 'pushbut-
ton','units','normalized', 'String',
'OPEN','Position', [0.06 0.44 0.05 0.04],...
    'Callback',
'GUI_hyperspectral_fun(7)','BackgroundColor',colo
r2);
```

Fig. 4.7 Graphs of $\delta_S(i)$ as well as $\delta_{CON}(i)$, $\delta_{ENE}(i)$ and $\delta_{HOM}(i)$ as a function of wavelength and (*black line*) the manually set threshold p_q

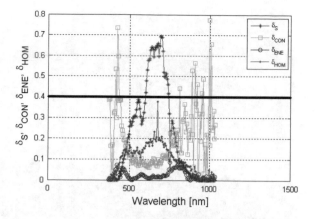

Fig. 4.8 Graph of changes in the mean, minimum and maximum brightness for the reference $L_S^W(i)$

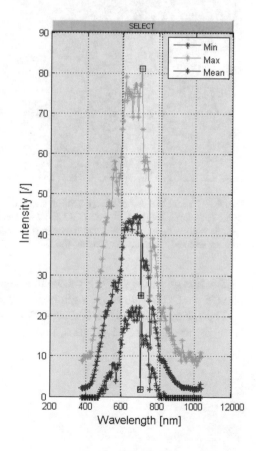

Figure 4.7 shows the graphs of $\delta_S(i)$ as well as $\delta_{CON}(i)$, $\delta_{ENE}(i)$ and $\delta_{HOM}(i)$ as a function of wavelength, whereas Fig. 4.8 shows a graph of changes in the mean, minimum and maximum brightness values for the reference $L_S^W(i)$.

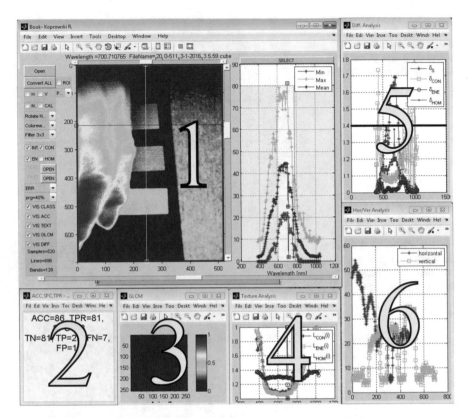

Fig. 4.9 The main menu of the application and additional windows: *1* main menu; *2* the results of *ACC*, *TPR*, *SPC*, *TN*, *TP*, *FN*, *FP*; *3* GLCM; *4* graphs of $L_{CON}(i)$, $L_{ENE}(i)$ and $L_{HOM}(i)$; *5* graphs of $\delta_S(i)$ as well as $\delta_{CON}(i)$, $\delta_{ENE}(i)$ and $\delta_{HOM}(i)$; *6* changes in the brightness for the *m*th row and *n*th column selected manually by moving the slider

The first graph (Fig. 4.7) is shown in a separate application window. The second one (Fig. 4.8) constitutes the right part of the main window—Fig. 4.9.

The values of *ACC*, *TPR*, *SPC*, *TN*, *TP*, *FN*, *FP* are calculated using the function GUI_hyperspectral_class, i.e.:

```
function
[ACC,TP,TN,FP,FN,TPR,SPC,meas,measT,nam,TRR]=GUI_hyper
spectral_class(diff_test_reference,wavelength_referenc
e_test,rect,prg,type)
...
global hObj

err=[diff_test_reference(:,1)];
meas=[];
measT=[];
nam=[];
TRR=(err(:,1)>rect(1))&(err(:,1)<rect(2));

if get(hObj(30),'Value')==1
    err=[err,diff_test_reference(:,2)];
    meas=[meas,wavelength_reference_test(:,2)];
    measT=[measT,wavelength_reference_test(:,6)];
    nam{length(nam)+1}='L_{INT}(i)';
end
if get(hObj(31),'Value')==1
    err=[err,diff_test_reference(:,3)];
    meas=[meas,wavelength_reference_test(:,3)];
    measT=[measT,wavelength_reference_test(:,7)];
    nam{length(nam)+1}='L_{CON}(i)';
end
if get(hObj(32),'Value')==1
    err=[err,diff_test_reference(:,4)];
    meas=[meas,wavelength_reference_test(:,4)];
    measT=[measT,wavelength_reference_test(:,8)];
    nam{length(nam)+1}='L_{ENE}(i)';
end
if get(hObj(33),'Value')==1
    err=[err,diff_test_reference(:,5)];
    meas=[meas,wavelength_reference_test(:,5)];
    measT=[measT,wavelength_reference_test(:,9)];
    nam{length(nam)+1}='L_{HOM}(i)';
end
if size(err,2)>=2;
    if type==1

err=[err,sum(err(:,2:end)>prg,2)>0,(err(:,1)>rect(1))&
(err(:,1)<rect(2))];
        TP=sum( (err(:,end-1)==1).*(err(:,end)==1) );
        TN=sum( (err(:,end-1)==0).*(err(:,end)==0) );
        FP=sum( (err(:,end-1)==1).*(err(:,end)==0) );
        FN=sum( (err(:,end-1)==0).*(err(:,end)==1) );
        ACC=round( (TP+TN)/(TP+TN+FP+FN).*100);
        TPR=round(TP/(TP+FN)*100);
        SPC=round(TN/(TN+FP)*100);
...
```

When analysing the next fragments of the proposed source code, it is divided into two areas:

- in the first area the values are gathered in the variable `err` constituting the basis for further analysis. Gathering is directly related to manual (by the user) determination which features ($\delta_S(i)$ as well as $\delta_{CON}(i)$, $\delta_{ENE}(i)$ and $\delta_{HOM}(i)$) are taken into account in the analysis. This option is provided by a suitable code fragment in the `GUI_hyperspectral`, i.e.:

```
hObj(30) =uicontrol('Style',
'checkbox','units','normalized', 'String',
'INT','Position', [0.01 0.57 0.05 0.05],...

'Callback','GUI_hyperspectral_fun(8)','Background
Color',color2,'Value',1);
hObj(31)=uicontrol('Style',
'checkbox','units','normalized', 'String',
'CON','Position', [0.051 0.57 0.059 0.05],...

'Callback','GUI_hyperspectral_fun(8)','Background
Color',color2);
hObj(32)=uicontrol('Style',
'checkbox','units','normalized', 'String',
'ENE','Position', [0.01 0.52 0.05 0.05],...

'Callback','GUI_hyperspectral_fun(8)','Background
Color',color2);
hObj(33)=uicontrol('Style',
'checkbox','units','normalized', 'String',
'HOM','Position', [0.051 0.52 0.059 0.05],...

'Callback','GUI_hyperspectral_fun(8)','Background
Color',color2);
```

When appropriate values (as selected) are added to the variable `err`, there follows its binarization with the threshold p_{rg} `sum(err(:,2:end) > prg,2) > 0`. Then the range of *TP* and *TN* located in the manually selected *ROI* is calculated, i.e.: `(err(:,1) > rect(1))&(err(:,1) < rect(2))`.

- In the other area, the values of *ACC, TPR, SPC, TN, TP, FN, FP* are calculated. The obtained results are shown in a separate window—Fig. 4.9 (2).

Depending on the option *INT, ENE, VAR, HOM* (Fig. 4.10) chosen to calculate *ACC, TPR, SPC, TN, TP, FN, FP*, different configurations of features are taken into account. Therefore, for the set threshold p_{rg} (in this case equal to 15%), different results are obtained. For example, for the *test* and *reference ROIs* shown in Fig. 4.11, the results for different configurations of features are presented in

Fig. 4.10 Fragment of the main menu with the elements responsible for image pre-processing—*green* and image processing—*red*: *1* calculation of intensity; *2* calculation of energy; *3* types of analysis *ERR/DEC TREE/BAYES/DISC/SVM*; *4* threshold p_{rg}; *5* on/off window of classification results; *6* on/off window of results of *ACC, TPR, SPC, TN, TP, FN, FP*; *7* on/off window of texture analysis; *8* on/off window of GLCM; *9* on/off window of graphs of feature errors; *10* choice of test/pattern analysis; *11* calculation of contrast; *12* calculation of homogeneity; *13* loading of the external file *test.mat*; *14* loading of the external file *reference.mat*

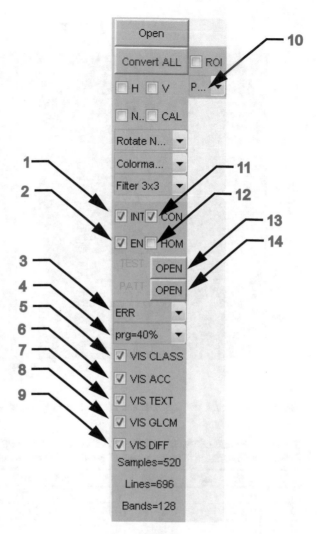

Table 4.2. The task is to verify the quality of the recognition of the skin area for a selected characteristic spectral region—Fig. 4.11 (right). In this case, 86 measurements of *TN* and 42 measurements of *TP* are marked. The number of measurements is equivalent to the number *I* of images for individual wavelengths.

Table 4.2 shows that the presented simple method of analysis of features does not work in every case. First, the results of *TPR, SPC* obtained for individual features (*INT, ENE, VAR* or *HOM*) are at the level of 0 and 100% or 0 and 87% (for *TPR* and *SPC* respectively). Secondly, in the present case, the feature which is brightness (*INT*) improves the results regardless of the presence of the other features

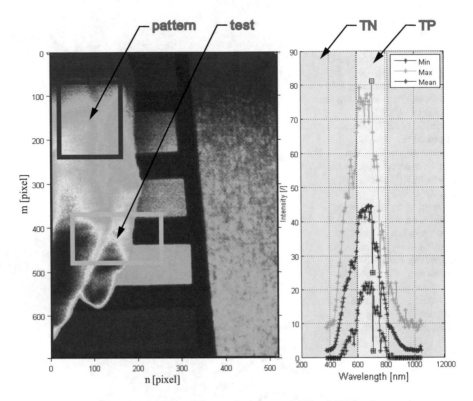

Fig. 4.11 *Reference* and *test ROIs* and the marked range of *TN* and *TP* for the tested case

Table 4.2 Results of *TN, TP, FN, FP* as well as *ACC, TPR, SPC* (expressed as a percentage) for different configurations of features—on/off position of checkbox objects (*INT, ENE, VAR, HOM*)[a]

INT	CON	ENE	HOM	ACC	TPR	SPC	TN	TP	FN	FP
0	0	0	1	67	0	100	86	0	42	0
0	0	1	0	67	0	100	86	0	42	0
0	0	1	1	67	0	100	86	0	42	0
0	1	0	0	59	0	87	75	0	42	11
0	1	0	1	59	0	87	75	0	42	11
0	1	1	0	59	0	87	75	0	42	11
0	1	1	1	59	0	87	75	0	42	11
1	0	0	0	90	69	100	86	29	13	0
1	0	0	1	90	69	100	86	29	13	0
1	0	1	0	90	69	100	86	29	13	0
1	0	1	1	90	69	100	86	29	13	0
1	1	0	0	81	69	87	75	29	13	11
1	1	0	1	81	69	87	75	29	13	11
1	1	1	0	81	69	87	75	29	13	11
1	1	1	1	81	69	87	75	29	13	11

[a]The value of '0' means that the feature does not occur, '1' that it occurs in calculations

(see the last rows in Table 4.2), i.e.: $TPR = 69\%$ and $SPC = 100\%$. To sum up, this simple method of analysis of features cannot use the full potential and results obtained from texture analysis. Consequently, the selected types of classifiers described in the following sections were implemented.

4.4   Block Diagram of the Discussed Transformations

The discussed transformations, extraction of features, including the parts of the source code are presented in the form of a block diagram in Fig. 4.12. This diagram applies to parts of the algorithm responsible for fundamental analysis of features. Additionally, it was subdivided into the part responsible for the extraction of features. The blocks of image acquisition and pre-processing have been discussed in earlier chapters of the monograph.

The block diagram will be further supplemented by the blocks associated with classification. The diagram intentionally does not include the module, the portion of the source code and the corresponding functionality of tracking changes in the contour, which, as mentioned above, readers can implement themselves.

The collected features are the basis for the construction of classifiers.

4.5   Measurement of Additional Features

The previous chapter discusses the features obtained from the analysis and processing of hyperspectral images, and to be more specific, derived from GLCM analysis of the *ROI* selected by the user. This analysis has been implemented in the described software both in terms of the source codes and the GUI. However, this is not the only possible implementation as well as not the only possible set of features. Typical analyses of textures used for hyperspectral images include: quadtree decomposition, Hough transform, entropy and not discussed above—correlation—extracted from the GLCM. Acquisition of these new features from the *ROI* is almost intuitive, and requires only the knowledge and the correct use of the function hough, entropy and the parameter of the function graycoprops which is 'Correlation'. Acquisition of quantitative scalar features from quadtree decomposition requires the use of qtdecomp and the following code implemented for:

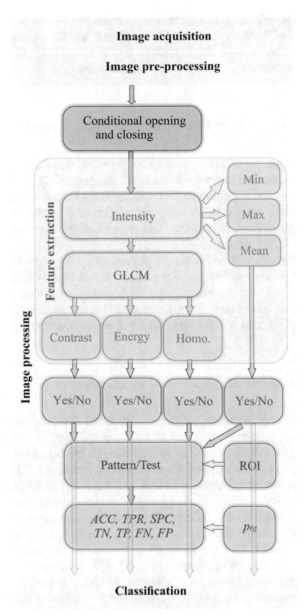

Fig. 4.12 Block diagram of the algorithm part responsible for fundamental analysis of features. The block diagram is subdivided into a part responsible for the extraction of the features. Blocks of image acquisition and pre-processing have been discussed in earlier chapters of the monograph. This diagram includes one of the blocks highlighted in *blue* whose functionality has not been included in the main application

```
L1=load('D:/k/_I20_L0-511_13-1-
2016_13.5.59.cube50.mat');
Lgray=mat2gray(L1.L1);
Lgray=imresize(Lgray,[512 512]);
figure; imshow(Lgray)
L2 = qtdecomp(Lgray,.27);
L3 = zeros(size(L2));
pam=[];
for q=0:9
  pam=[pam;[2^q length(find(L2==2^q))]];
  if pam(end,2)>0
    L4=ones([2^q 2^q pam(end,2)]);
    L4(2:2^q,2:2^q,:)=0;
    L3=qtsetblk(L3,L2,2^q,L4);
  end
end
L3(end,1:end)=1;
L3(1:end,end)=1;
L5=Lgray; L5(L3==1)=1;
figure, imshow(L5,[]);
xlabel('n
[pixel]','FontSize',14,'FontAngle','Italic');
ylabel('m [pixel]','FontSize',14,'FontAngle','Italic')
figure; plot(pam(:,1),pam(:,2),'-r*'); hold on; grid
on
xlabel('N_q=M_q
[pixel]','FontSize',14,'FontAngle','Italic');
ylabel('number of blocks [/]','FontSize',14);
```

The presented source code contains a loop that enables to change the size of the sought areas (q=0:9 for a code fragment find(L2==2^q)). If at least one area of this size (if pam(end,2)>0) is found, it is filled with blocks:

```
L4=ones([2^q 2^q pam(end,2)]);
L4(2:2^q,2:2^q,:)=0;
```

The results obtained for the threshold above which the division into smaller blocks was performed, i.e.: $p_{qt} = 0.27$, is shown in Figs. 4.13 and 4.14.

Figure 4.13 shows the image $L_{GRAY}(m, n, i)$ with a superimposed division into individual blocks sized from $M_q \times N_q = 1 \times 1$ pixel to $M_q \times N_q = 512 \times 512$ pixels. The size of each block is a power of 2, i.e.: it is equal to 2^q for $q \in (0, 10)$ for the analysed case. Attention should be paid here to the need to resize the image $L_{GRAY}(m, n, i)$ to the size of rows and columns that are a power of two. Figure 4.14 shows a graph of the total number of blocks $M_q \times N_q$ as a function of

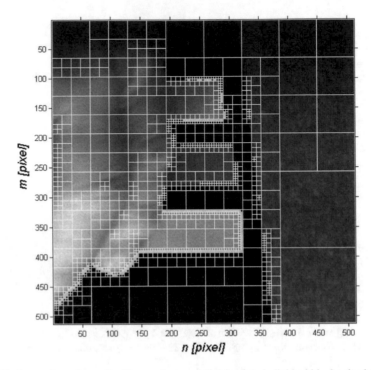

Fig. 4.13 Image $L_{GRAY}(m, n, i)$ with superimposed division into individual blocks sized $M_q \times N_q$

Fig. 4.14 Graph of the total
number of blocks as a
function of their size
$M_q \times N_q$

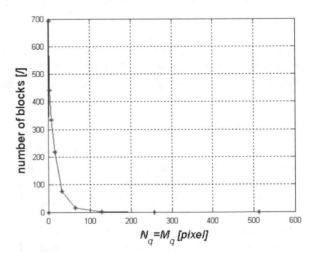

their size. This type of analysis can complement the existing analysis presented in the previous chapters. It may also be carried out for all i images of the sequence (for different wavelengths). In this case (analysis of an image sequence for $i \in (1, 128)$), the source code has been modified to the following form:

```
pam=[];hObj=waitbar(0,'Please wait...');
for i=1:128
    L1=load(['D:/k/_I20_L0-511_13-1-
2016_13.5.59.cube',mat2str(i),'.mat']);
    Lgray=mat2gray(L1.L1);
    Lgray=imresize(Lgray,[512 512]);
    L2 = qtdecomp(Lgray,.27);
    L3 = zeros(size(L2));
    for d=0:9
        pam(i,d+1)=length(find(L2==2^d));
    end
waitbar(i/128)
end
close(hObj)
figure, mesh(pam);
xlabel('q+1
[pixel]','FontSize',14,'FontAngle','Italic');
ylabel('i [/]','FontSize',14,'FontAngle','Italic');
zlabel('number of blocks
[/]','FontSize',14,'FontAngle','Italic');
figure, plot(pam(:,1),'-r*'); hold on; grid on
xlabel('i [/]','FontSize',14,'FontAngle','Italic');
ylabel('number of blocks
[/]','FontSize',14,'FontAngle','Italic')
```

As is apparent from the above source code, the said modification involves the introduction of automatic analysis of all images of the sequence ($i \in (1, 128)$), and plotting, at the end of the algorithm, a graph. The results obtained are shown in Figs. 4.15 and 4.16.

Figure 4.15 shows a graph of changes in the number of blocks sized $M_q \times N_q$ as a function of their size for subsequent i images. As is apparent from the presented graph, the number of the smallest areas sized $M_q \times N_q = 1 \times 1$ pixel is the greatest for each i image. Figure 4.16 shows a graph of the total number of blocks sized $M_q \times N_q = 1 \times 1$ pixel as a function of subsequent i images.

The above are excerpts of the code of *m-files* GUI_hyperspectral_qtdecomp_test and GUI_hyperspectral_qtdecomp_test2 that are available to the reader in the form of supporting materials attached to this monograph.

Apart from the discussed features that can be analysed, other calculations can also be performed. New features can be obtained from image analysis using

Fig. 4.15 Graph of changes
in the number of blocks sized
$M_q \times N_q$ as a function of their
size (2^q) for subsequent
i images

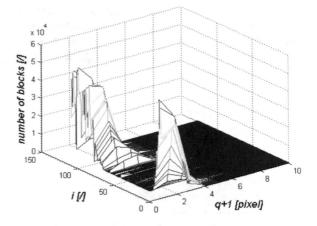

Fig. 4.16 Graph of the total
number of blocks sized
$M_q \times N_q = 1 \times 1$ pixel as a
function of subsequent
i images

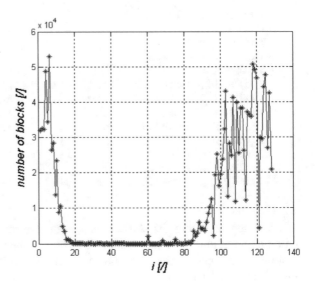

Riesz transform [5–7] or Gabor filtration. The basis will be a Gaussian function for
three dimensions [8–10], i.e.:

$$h_{GA}(m_{GA}, n_{GA}, i_{GA}, \sigma_m, \sigma_n, \sigma_i)$$
$$= A_{GA} \times \exp\left(-\frac{m_{GA}^2}{2 \times \sigma_m^2} - \frac{n_{GA}^2}{2 \times \sigma_n^2} - \frac{i_{GA}^2}{2 \times \sigma_i^2}\right) \qquad (4.23)$$

where

$$A_{GA} = \frac{1}{\sigma_m \times \sigma_n \times \sigma_i \times (2 \times \pi)^{\frac{3}{2}}} \tag{4.24}$$

and σ_m, σ_n, σ_i—standard deviation of the mean for three dimensions m, n, i.

m_{GA}, n_{GA}, i_{GA}—values m, n, i normalized to the range from -0.5 to 0.5, for example for m_{GA}:

$$m_{GA} = \frac{m}{M} - 0.5 \tag{4.25}$$

Due to the nature of hyperspectral images of the skin, in practice, it is often necessary to rotate the mask h_{GA} but only in two dimensions, i.e. the new coordinates $(m_{GA\theta}, n_{GA\theta})$ after rotation are equal (similarly to Sect. 3.1. Affine transformations of the image):

$$m_{GA\theta} = -m_{GA} \times \sin(\theta) + n_{GA} \times \cos(\theta) \tag{4.26}$$

$$n_{GA\theta} = n_{GA} \times \cos(\theta) + m_{GA} \times \sin(\theta) \tag{4.27}$$

Also in practical applications [11–16], it is often necessary to use a derivative in each of the three possible dimensions. Therefore, it was assumed, for simplicity of calculations, that the variable h_{devGA} will be the result of calculating the derivative in three dimensions. The superscript will mean the wth degree of the derivative for three consecutive dimensions. For example, $h_{devGA}^{(0,0,1)}$ is the first derivative in the third dimension, i.e.:

$$h_{devGA}^{(0,0,1)}(m_{GA\theta}, n_{GA\theta}, i_{GA\theta}, \sigma_m, \sigma_n, \sigma_i) = \frac{\partial h_{GA}(m_{GA\theta}, n_{GA\theta}, i_{GA\theta}, \sigma_m, \sigma_n, \sigma_i)}{\partial i_{GA}} \tag{4.28}$$

On this basis, it is possible to create a pyramid of masks h_{devGA} for changes in various arguments. Changes in the angle θ in the range $\theta \in (0, 2 \cdot \pi)$, e.g. every value of 0.1, are most often used. The results obtained in the form of a pyramid of masks h_{devGA} are shown in Fig. 4.17.

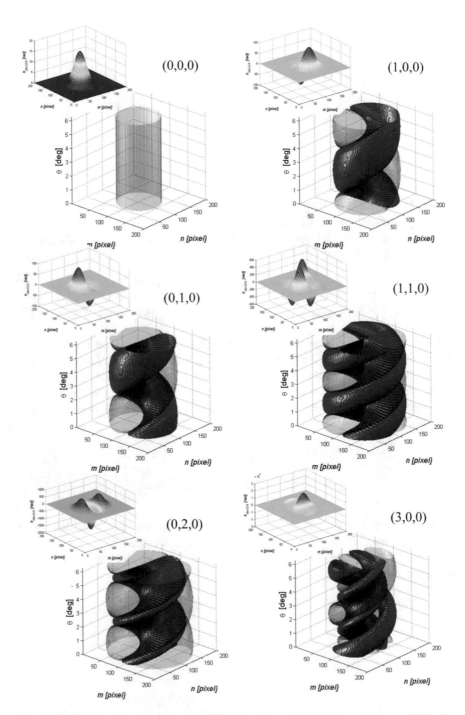

Fig. 4.17 Pyramid of masks h_{devGA} for $\theta \in (0, 2 \cdot \pi)$ every 0.1 and various degrees of derivatives $h_{devGA}^{(0,0,0)}, h_{devGA}^{(1,0,0)}, h_{devGA}^{(1,1,0)}, h_{devGA}^{(1,1,1)}, h_{devGA}^{(2,0,0)}$ and $h_{devGA}^{(0,2,1)}$. Negative values of the mask are marked in *red*, and positive values in *blue*. In each case, one of the masks for $\theta = 0°$ has been placed in the *top left corner*

The masks h_{devGA} shown in Fig. 4.17 were calculated for $\theta \in (0,2\cdot\pi)$ every 0.1 and various degrees of derivatives $h_{devGA}^{(0,0,0)}$, $h_{devGA}^{(1,0,0)}$, $h_{devGA}^{(1,1,0)}$, $h_{devGA}^{(1,1,1)}$, $h_{devGA}^{(2,0,0)}$ and $h_{devGA}^{(0,2,1)}$. Negative values of the mask are marked in red (Fig. 4.17), and positive values in blue. These results were obtained using two functions. The first one is dergauss which calculates the derivative of the Gaussian function for the row $w \in (0, 4)$, i.e.:

```
function y = dergauss(x,sigma,w)
if w==0
    y = exp(-x.^2/(2*sigma^2)) / (sigma*sqrt(2*pi));
elseif w==1
    y =(-x./(sigma.^2)).*exp(-x.^2/(2.*sigma.^2)) ./
(sigma.*sqrt(2.*pi));
elseif w==2
    y =((x.^2-sigma.^2)./(sigma.^4)).*exp(-
x.^2/(2.*sigma.^2)) ./ (sigma.*sqrt(2.*pi));
elseif w==3
    y =( (x.^3-3.*x.*sigma.^2) ./(sigma.^6)).*exp(-
x.^2/(2.*sigma.^2)) ./ (sigma.*sqrt(2.*pi));
elseif w==4
    y =( (x.^4-
6.*x.^2.*sigma.^2+3.*sigma.^4)./(sigma.^8)).*exp(-
x.^2/(2.*sigma.^2)) ./ (sigma.*sqrt(2.*pi));
else
end
```

As is apparent from the presented function, for each condition (the degree of derivative—the value of the variable w), the value of y is calculated using a different formula.

The second function is Gauss_test with the following source code:

```
hdevGA=[];
sigman=0.1;
sigmam=0.1;
M=200;N=200;
devm=3;
devn=0;
hObj = waitbar(0,'Please wait...');
for theta=0:0.1:(2*pi);
    [nGA,mGA]=meshgrid(linspace(-0.5,0.5,M),linspace(-
0.5,0.5,N));
    nGAtheta=nGA.*cos(theta)+mGA.*sin(theta);
    mGAtheta=-nGA.*sin(theta)+mGA.*cos(theta);
hdevGA(1:M,1:N,round(theta*10+1))=dergauss(nGAtheta,si
gman,devn).*dergauss(mGAtheta,sigmam,devm);
    if theta ==0
        figure; mesh(hdevGA)
        xlabel('m
[pixel]','FontSize',14,'FontAngle','Italic')
        ylabel('n
[pixel]','FontSize',14,'FontAngle','Italic')
        zlabel('h_{devGA}
[rad]','FontSize',14,'FontAngle','Italic')
    end

    waitbar(theta/(2*pi),hObj)
end
close(hObj)
figure
[n,m,i]=meshgrid( 1:size(hdevGA,2) , 1:size(hdevGA,1)
, 0:0.1:(2*pi));
p1 =
patch(isosurface(n,m,i,hdevGA>1,0.1),'FaceColor',[0 0
1 ],'EdgeColor','none');
alpha(p1,0.2)
p2 = patch(isosurface(n,m,i,hdevGA<-
1,0.1),'FaceColor',[1 0 0 ],'EdgeColor','none');
alpha(p2,0.9)
view(41,24);
camlight; camlight(-80,-10); lighting phong;
grid on
hold on
axis square
axis([1 N 1 M 0 2*pi])
xlabel('m [pixel]','FontSize',14,'FontAngle','Italic')
ylabel('n [pixel]','FontSize',14,'FontAngle','Italic')
zlabel('\theta  [deg]','FontSize',14)
```

The first part of this source code relates to the declaration of variables and determination of their values. Then the values of matrices nGA, mGA are determined, which are the basis for calculating the mask h_{devGA}. Rotation by the angle theta is initially implemented. In the next step, the previously discussed function dergauss is used. In the final stage, a three-dimensional graph (Fig. 4.17) is shown using the functions patch and isosurface.

The results of the presented functions (dergauss, Gauss_test) are shown in Fig. 4.17, but this is only one of many cases of the pyramid. In hyperspectral imaging the derivative in the third axis is also often used for analysis and acquisition of features (the results shown earlier involve only two axes and rotation). The function dergauss will be still used as well as the following new command sequence Gauss_test2:

```
hdevGA=[];
sigman=0.08;
sigmam=0.08;
sigmai=0.08;
devm=2;
devn=0;
devi=0;
M=100;N=100;I=100;
Ii=linspace(-0.5,0.5,I);
Iid=dergauss(Ii,sigmai,devi);
hObj = waitbar(0,'Please wait...');
for i=1:length(Iid);
    [nGA,mGA]=meshgrid(linspace(-0.5,0.5,M),linspace(-
0.5,0.5,N));

hdevGA(1:M,1:N,i)=dergauss(nGA,sigman,devn).*dergauss(
mGA,sigmam,devm).*Iid(i);
    waitbar(i/length(Iid),hObj)
end

close(hObj)
figure
[n,m,i]=meshgrid( 1:size(hdevGA,2) , 1:size(hdevGA,1)
, 1:size(hdevGA,3));
p1 =
patch(isosurface(n,m,i,hdevGA>1,0.1),'FaceColor',[0 0
1 ],'EdgeColor','none');
alpha(p1,0.9)
p2 = patch(isosurface(n,m,i,hdevGA<-
1,0.1),'FaceColor',[1 0 0 ],'EdgeColor','none');
alpha(p2,0.9)
view(41,24);
camlight; camlight(-80,-10); lighting phong;
grid on
hold on
axis square
axis([1 N 1 M 0 length(Iid)])
xlabel('m [pixel]','FontSize',14,'FontAngle','Italic')
ylabel('n [pixel]','FontSize',14,'FontAngle','Italic')
zlabel('i [pixel]','FontSize',14,'FontAngle','Italic')
```

As in the previously discussed source code, the values of constants are initially declared along with 3D spaces of variable parameters ([nGA,mGA]=mesh-grid...). Next, for subsequent i, values of hdevGA(1:M,1:N,i) are declared. In the last stage, the results in three dimensional space are shown. They are presented in Fig. 4.18.

The results in Fig. 4.18 indicate the range of variation in the masks h_{devGA} with respect to different degrees of derivatives for three dimensions. Other parameters that can be changed for individual dimensions are θ and σ. Figure 4.19 shows different variants of a sequence of masks for different values of the degree of derivatives, and various values of standard deviations of the mean σ. The following is a portion of the source code that was used to create Fig. 4.19, i.e.:

```
hdevGA=[];
sigman=0.01;
sigmam=0.18;
sigmai=0.08;
devm=0;
devn=1;
devi=2;
M=100;N=100;I=100;
Ii=linspace(-0.5,0.5,I);
Iid=dergauss(Ii,sigmai,devi);
hObj = waitbar(0,'Please wait...');
for i=1:length(Iid);
    [nGA,mGA]=meshgrid(linspace(-0.5,0.5,M),linspace(-
0.5,0.5,N));
    theta=i/I*pi;
    nGAtheta=nGA.*cos(theta)+mGA.*sin(theta);
    mGAtheta=-nGA.*sin(theta)+mGA.*cos(theta);

hdevGA(1:M,1:N,i)=dergauss(nGAtheta,sigman,devn).*derg
auss(mGAtheta,sigmam,devm).*Iid(i);
    waitbar(i/length(Iid),hObj)
end
```

Masks h_{devGA} defined for different values of parameters enable to acquire features that are not available for typical methods of analysis and typical known mask filters (Sobel, Roberts or Canny). This problem is visible for simple binarization of a sequence of images $L_{GRAY}(m, n, i)$ for two thresholds equal to 0.5 (Fig. 4.20—red) and 0.4 (Fig. 4.20—blue).

The results of the convolution of the image $L_{GRAY}(m, n, i)$ with the pyramid of masks $h_{devGA}{}^{(1,0,0)}$, $\theta = 0°$ and $\sigma = 0.08$ (see Fig. 4.18), are shown in Fig. 4.21. The colours (Fig. 4.21) indicate the results of binarization for the negative areas (blue) and positive ones (red). The acquisition of a feature from each ith image, necessary

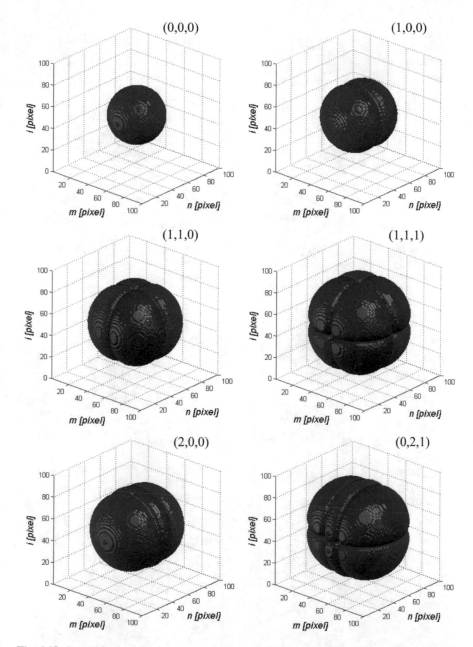

Fig. 4.18 Pyramid of masks h_{devGA} for three dimensions and different degrees of derivatives $h_{devGA}^{(0,0,0)}, h_{devGA}^{(1,0,0)}, h_{devGA}^{(1,1,0)}, h_{devGA}^{(1,1,1)}, h_{devGA}^{(2,0,0)}$ and $h_{devGA}^{(0,2,1)}$ (respectively) when $\theta = 0°$ and $\sigma = 0.08$. Negative values of the mask are marked in *red*, and the positive ones in *blue*

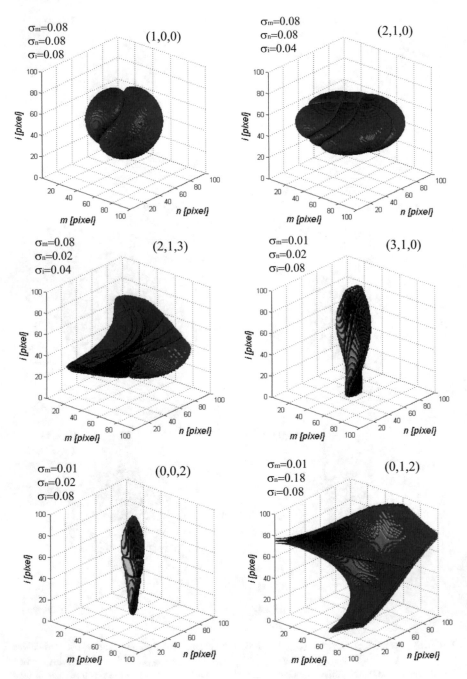

Fig. 4.19 Pyramid of masks h_{devGA} for three dimensions, different degrees of derivatives and various values of σ. Negative values of the mask are marked in *red*, and the positive ones in *blue*

Fig. 4.20 Results of
binarization of the image
$L_{GRAY}(m, n, i)$ for two
thresholds equal to 0.5 (*red*)
and 0.4 (*blue*)

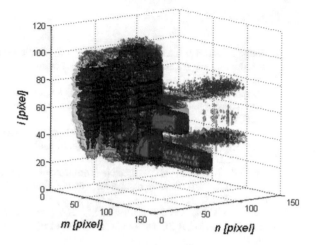

Fig. 4.21 Result of the
convolution of the image
$L_{GRAY}(m, n, i)$ with the
pyramid of masks $h_{devGA}^{(1,0,0)}$,
$\theta = 0°$ and $\sigma = 0.08$ (see
Fig. 4.18). The *colours*
indicate the results of
binarization for the negative
areas (*blue*) and positive ones
(*red*)

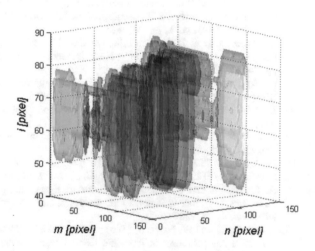

for further use in the classification, is dependent on the type of the processing task. This can be either the maximum or minimum value of the image convolution $L_{CONV}(m, n, i)$ (Fig. 4.21), as well as the surface area of the areas above or below the predetermined threshold. As mentioned earlier, pyramids of masks h_{devGA} are generally profiled to a specific type of images and their nature. This applies to both hyperspectral images and other types of medical images.

The final parts of the source code are in the *m-files* `Gauss_test3` and `Gauss_test4` and are available as supplementary material attached to this monograph.

References

1. Quinzán I, Sotoca JM, Latorre-Carmona P, Pla F, García-Sevilla P, Boldó E., Band selection in spectral imaging for non-invasive melanoma diagnosis. Biomed Opt Express. 2013 Apr 1;4 (4):514–9

2. Qi B, Zhao C, Youn E, Nansen C. Use of weighting algorithms to improve traditional support vector machine based classifications of reflectance data. Opt Express. 2011 Dec 19;19 (27):26816–26

3. Hennessy R, Bish S, Tunnell JW, Markey MK. Segmentation of diffuse reflectance hyperspectral datasets with noise for detection of Melanoma. Conf Proc IEEE Eng Med Biol Soc. 2012;2012:1482–5.

4. Chen TF, Baranoski GV. Effective compression and reconstruction of human skin hyperspectral reflectance databases. Conf Proc IEEE Eng Med Biol Soc. 2015 Aug;2015:7027–30.

5. D. Van De Ville, N. Chenouard and M. Unser, "Steerable Pyramids and Tight Wavelet Frames in L2(ℝd)", IEEE Transactions on Image Processing, vol. 20, no. 10, pp. 2705–2721, October 2011.

6. E. Simoncelli and W. Freeman, "The steerable pyramid: A flexible architecture for multi-scale derivative computation," in Proceedings of the International Conference on Image Processing, Oct. 23–26, 1995, vol 3, pp. 444-447.

7. M. Unser, D. Sage, D. Van De Ville,"Multiresolution Monogenic Signal Analysis Using the Riesz-Laplace Wavelet Transform", IEEE Transactions on Image Processing, vol. 18, no. 11, pp. 2402–2418, November 2009.

8. M. Michaelis and G. Sommer, "A Lie group approach to steerable filters," Reference Recognit. Lett., vol. 16, no. 11, pp. 1165–1174, 1995.

9. Y. Hel-Or and P. C. Teo, "Canonical decomposition of steerable functions," J. Math. Imag. Vis., vol. 9, no. 1, pp. 83–95, 1998.

10. P. C. Teo and Y. Hel-Or, "Lie generators for computing steerable functions," Reference Recognit. Lett., vol. 19, no. 1, pp. 7–17, 1998.

11. E. P. Simoncelli, W. T. Freeman, E. H. Adelson, and D. J. Heeger, "Shiftable multiscale transforms," IEEE Trans. Inf. Theory, vol. 38, no. 2, pp. 587–607, 1992.

12. A. Karasaridis and E. Simoncelli, "A filter design technique for steerable pyramid image transforms," in Proc. IEEE Int. Conf. Acoustics, Speech, and Signal Processing, May 7–10, 1996, vol. 4, pp. 2387–2390.

13. E. Simoncelli and W. Freeman, "The steerable pyramid: a flexible architecture for multi-scale derivative computation," in Proc. Int. Conf. Image Processing, Oct. 23–26, 1995, vol. 3, pp. 444–447.

14. Y. Wiaux, L. Jacques, and P. Vandergheynst, "Correspondence principle between spherical and Euclidean wavelets," Astrophys. J., vol. 632, p. 15, 2005.

15. J. G. Daugman, "Complete discrete 2-D Gabor transforms by neural networks for image-analysis and compression," IEEE Trans. Acoust. Speech Signal Process., vol. 36, no. 7, pp. 1169–1179, Jul. 1988.

16. E. J. Candès and D. L. Donoho, "Ridgelets: A key to higher-dimensional intermittency?," Phil. Trans. Roy. Soc. Lond. A., pp. 2495–2509, 1999.

Chapter 5
Classification

The acquired image features such as mean brightness, contrast, energy and homogeneity can be used for machine learning and classification. Of the many types of classifiers, decision trees, the naive Bayes classifier, discriminant analysis and support vector machine were selected. The training mode for all classifiers is carried out in the same way. The group of data is a set of four features (brightness, contrast, energy and homogeneity) calculated for two *ROIs* selected by the user. **The first region**, whose data may be also loaded as a *reference.mat* file, relates to the training area. **The second ROI** concerns the test area, and the data on individual features can also be loaded from an external file *test.mat*. The length of the test and training data vectors is dependent on the user and the number of analysed i images. It is also dependent on the number of common, for both the training and test group, wavelengths. Each ith image complying with these conditions creates a new record in the training vector entering four subsequent scalar values. The idea of selecting the values *reference* and *test* and the *ROI* is shown schematically in Fig. 5.1.

Figure 5.1 shows a schematic diagram of an exemplary pattern and test vector created from the variables $L_S(i)$, $L_{CON}(i)$, $L_{ENE}(i)$ and $L_{HOM}(i)$. The results that are deleted are marked in red, whereas the results participating in training and testing the classifier in blue. The green area results from harmonisation, for each analysis, of common wavelengths. In this case, these are the values 900, 901, 902, 903 and 904 nm. The vectors (training and test) thus prepared are used in the construction and testing of the following classifiers (mentioned above):

- decision trees,
- naive Bayes classifier,
- discriminant analysis and
- support vector machine.

© Springer International Publishing AG 2017
R. Koprowski, *Processing of Hyperspectral Medical Images*,
Studies in Computational Intelligence 682,
DOI 10.1007/978-3-319-50490-2_5

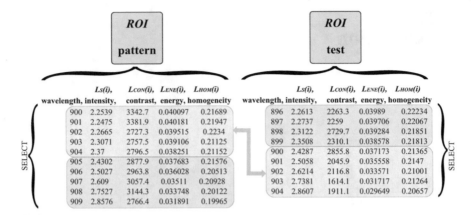

Fig. 5.1 Schematic diagram of an exemplary pattern and test vector created from the variables $L_S(i)$, $L_{CON}(i)$, $L_{ENE}(i)$ and $L_{HOM}(i)$. The results which are deleted are marked in *red*, and the results participating in training and testing the classifier in *blue*

These classifiers and their implementation are described in detail in the next subchapters (for this purpose Statistics Toolbox is additionally required). For the classifiers described in the following subchapters, the same test and pattern data were used. They were obtained from the manually selected areas of the image shown in Fig. 4.11. In total, 92 cases of wavelengths for which there should be compliance with the pattern and 36 cases where such compliance cannot exist were obtained for the test and training vectors.

The length of both vectors is due to the results of harmonisation of wavelengths (see Fig. 4.6). In this case, there was complete compatibility of wavelengths—the analysed *ROIs* come from the same image $L_{GRAY}(m, n, i)$.

5.1 Decision Trees

Decision trees have been used in machine learning [1] for many years [2–17]. They have been also used and implemented in Matlab for a few years. Several functions are designed for this purpose:

- `classregtree`—function responsible for the tree induction,
- `test`—function responsible for testing the tree,
- `prune`—function responsible for pruning the tree.

The Gini index is the criterion for assessing the split point of decision trees used in Matlab. Decision trees were induced using the CART algorithm. Classification with the use of decision trees was implemented in the function GUI_hyperspectral_class_dec_tree. This function can be divided into several areas. In the first area, the true and false cases were divided into 'Yes' and 'No' strings, i.e.:

```
function
[TP,TN,FP,FN,ACC,TPR,SPC]=GUI_hyperspectral_class_dec_
tree(TRR,meas,measT,nam)
...
global hObj
species=[];
for ijj=1:length(TRR)
    if TRR(ijj)==1
        species{ijj}='Yes';
    else
        species{ijj}='No';
    end
end
```

In the next area, the tree is induced and tested for the training data, i.e.:

```
tt = classregtree(meas, species','names',nam);
[cost,secost,ntermnodes,best]=test(tt,'cross',meas,spe
cies');
resubcost = test(tt,'resub');
```

In the next area, the tree is pruned.

```
pt = prune(tt,best);
```

The last part of the function refers to the visualization of both cross-validation and resubstitution and the site of tree pruning. 2D and 3D graphs are also shown depending on the number of features selected for analysis, i.e.:

```
if get(hObj(72),'Value')==1
    [mincost,minloc] = min(cost);
    cutoff = mincost + secost(minloc);
    figure;
    plot(ntermnodes,cost,'b-',
ntermnodes,resubcost,'r--')
    hold on; grid on
    plot([0 20], [cutoff cutoff], 'k:')
    plot(ntermnodes(best+1), cost(best+1), 'mo')
    legend('Cross-validation','Resubstitution','Min +
1 std. err.','Best choice')
    hold off
    view(tt);
    view(pt);
end
[grpname,~] = pt.eval(measT);
TP=sum( strcmp(grpname,'Yes').* strcmp(species','Yes')
); %
TN=sum( strcmp(grpname,'No') .* strcmp(species','No')
); %
FN=sum( strcmp(grpname,'No') .* strcmp(species','Yes')
); %
FP=sum( strcmp(grpname,'Yes').* strcmp(species','No')
); %
ACC= round((TP+TN)/(FN+FP+TN+TP).*100);
TPR= round(TP/(TP+FN).*100);
SPC= round(TN/(TN+FP).*100);
if get(hObj(72),'Value')==1
    if size(measT,2)==2
        figure;
plot(measT(strcmp(species','Yes'),1),measT(strcmp(spec
ies','Yes'),2),'r*'); hold on

plot(measT(strcmp(species','No'),1),measT(strcmp(speci
es','No'),2),'g*');

plot(measT(strcmp(grpname,'Yes'),1),measT(strcmp(grpna
me,'Yes'),2),'rs');

plot(measT(strcmp(grpname,'No'),1),measT(strcmp(grpnam
e,'No'),2),'gs'); grid on
        xlabel(nam{1},'FontSize',16);
        ylabel(nam{2},'FontSize',16);
        legend('Positive-expert','Negative-
expert','Positive-test','Negative-test')
    end
    if size(measT,2)>2
        figure;
```

```
plot3(measT(strcmp(species','Yes'),1),measT(strcmp(spe
cies','Yes'),2),measT(strcmp(species','Yes'),3),'r*');
hold on

plot3(measT(strcmp(species','No'),1),measT(strcmp(spec
ies','No'),2),measT(strcmp(species','No'),3),'g*');

plot3(measT(strcmp(grpname,'Yes'),1),measT(strcmp(grpn
ame,'Yes'),2),measT(strcmp(grpname,'Yes'),3),'rs');

plot3(measT(strcmp(grpname,'No'),1),measT(strcmp(grpna
me,'No'),2),measT(strcmp(grpname,'No'),3),'gs'); grid
on
        xlabel(nam{1},'FontSize',16);
        ylabel(nam{2},'FontSize',16);
        zlabel(nam{3},'FontSize',16);
        % surface
        LI=100;
        [x,y,z]=meshgrid( lin-
space(min(measT(:,1)),max(measT(:,1)),100) , lin-
space(min(measT(:,2)),max(measT(:,2)),100)
,linspace(min(measT(:,3)),max(measT(:,3)),100));
        X = x(:); Y = y(:); Z=z(:);
        [v,~] = pt.eval([X Y Z]);
        v=reshape(v,LI,LI,LI);
        p1 =
patch(isosurface(x,y,z,(strcmp(v,'Yes')),0.5),'FaceCol
or',[0 0 1 ],'EdgeColor','none');
        view(3); axis tight
        camlight; camlight(-80,-10); lighting phong;
        grid on
        alpha(p1,0.3)
        legend('Positive-expert','Negative-
expert','Positive-test','Negative-test')
        % end surface
    end
end
```

This function (GUI_hyperspectral_class_dec_tree) is activated by the function GUI_hyperspectral_class in one of the lines verifying the user's choice of a decision tree as a classifier, i.e.:

```
elseif type==2% Dec Tree

[TP,TN,FP,FN,ACC,TPR,SPC]=GUI_hyperspectral_class_dec_
tree(TRR,meas,measT,nam);
);
```

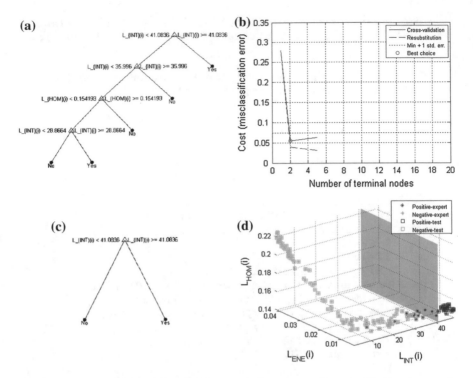

Fig. 5.2 Graphs of **a** the complete decision tree; **b** dependence of cross-validation errors on the number of tree nodes; **c** the pruned decision tree; **d** the results of classification

The decision trees thus implemented were tested for three features (brightness, energy, homogeneity) acquired from the *reference* and *test ROIs* shown in Fig. 4.11. The obtained results are presented in Fig. 5.2.

The graph presented in Fig. 5.2d and the pruned decision tree provide in this case: *ACC* = 88%, *TPR* = 56%, *SPC* = 100%, *TN* = 92, *TP* = 20, *FN* = 16 and *FP* = 0. Table 5.1 shows the results of *ACC*, *TPR*, *SPC*, *TN*, *TP*, *FN*, *FP* (expressed as a percentage) for various combinations of the features.

As is apparent from Table 5.1, brightness (*INT*) improves sensitivity to 56% compared to other combinations of features. In the case of the combinations of some of the features such as.: *HOM*, *ENE*, *ENE* and *HOM*, *CON* and *ENE*, *CON ENE* and *HOM*, *TPR* = 0%. Much better results are obtained in the case of the same data for another type of a classifier.

Table 5.1 Results of *TN*, *TP*, *FN*, *FP* as well as *ACC*, *TPR*, *SPC* (expressed as a percentage) for the pruned decision tree for different combinations of features—on/off position of checkbox objects (*INT*, *ENE*, *VAR*, *HOM*)[a]

INT	CON	ENE	HOM	ACC	TPR	SPC	TN	TP	FN	FP
0	0	0	1	66	0	92	85	0	36	7
0	0	1	0	72	0	100	92	0	36	0
0	0	1	1	72	0	100	92	0	36	0
0	1	0	0	75	11	100	92	4	32	0
0	1	0	1	75	11	100	92	4	32	0
0	1	1	0	72	0	100	92	0	36	0
0	1	1	1	72	0	100	92	0	36	0
1	0	0	0	88	56	100	92	20	16	0
1	0	0	1	88	56	100	92	20	16	0
1	0	1	0	88	56	100	92	20	16	0
1	0	1	1	88	56	100	92	20	16	0
1	1	0	0	88	56	100	92	20	16	0
1	1	0	1	88	56	100	92	20	16	0
1	1	1	0	88	56	100	92	20	16	0
1	1	1	1	88	56	100	92	20	16	0

[a]The value of '0' means that the feature does not occur, '1' that it occurs in calculations

5.2 Naive Bayes Classifier

One possible classification method implemented in MATLAB is a naive Bayes classifier [18–31]. It is based on the assumption of the mutual independence of the independent variables [19–21]. This simple probabilistic classifier provides good results in hyperspectral image classification. The implementation of the naive Bayes classifier [23–25] was carried out in the function `GUI_hyperspec-tral_class_naiv_bayes`. The greater part of the source code is the same as in the function `GUI_hyperspectral_class_dec_tree` for decision trees. The following shows only a portion of the source code for the most important differences between these functions, i.e.:

```
...
nbGau= NaiveBayes.fit(meas, species');
grpname= nbGau.predict(measT);
TP=sum( strcmp(grpname,'Yes').* strcmp(species','Yes')
); %
TN=sum( strcmp(grpname,'No') .* strcmp(species','No')
); %
FN=sum( strcmp(grpname,'No') .* strcmp(species','Yes')
); %
FP=sum( strcmp(grpname,'Yes').* strcmp(species','No')
); %
ACC= round((TP+TN)/(FN+FP+TN+TP).*100);
TPR= round(TP/(TP+FN).*100);
SPC= round(TN/(TN+FP).*100);
...
```

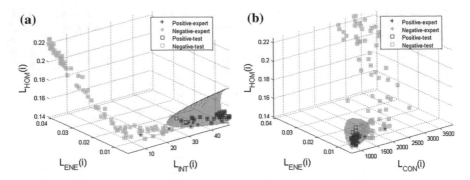

Fig. 5.3 Results of classification with a naive Bayes classifier. Negative and positive cases (wavelengths) are marked in *green* and *red* and the classification function in *blue*: **a** for features: intensity ($L_{INT}(i)$), homogeneity ($L_{HOM}(i)$) and energy ($L_{ENE}(i)$); **b** for features: contrast ($L_{CON}(i)$), homogeneity ($L_{HOM}(i)$) and energy ($L_{ENE}(i)$)

The results of classification, for the same training and test data as in the case of decision trees described in the previous subchapter (for the test and training vectors, 92 cases of wavelengths for which there should be compliance with the pattern and 36 cases where such compliance cannot exist), are shown in Fig. 5.3 and Table 5.2.

As follows from the numerical values in Table 5.2, the highest value of $ACC = 94\%$ was obtained for the combination of features INT and ENE. The smallest value of $ACC = 66\%$ was obtained for a single feature HOM.

Table 5.2 Results of TN, TP, FN, FP as well as ACC, TPR, SPC (expressed as a percentage) for the nave Bayes classifier for different combinations of features—on/off position of checkbox objects (INT, ENE, VAR, HOM)[a]

INT	CON	ENE	HOM	ACC	TPR	SPC	TN	TP	FN	FP
0	0	0	1	66	25	83	76	9	27	16
0	0	1	0	92	89	93	86	32	4	6
0	0	1	1	84	69	90	83	25	11	9
0	1	0	0	85	61	95	87	22	14	5
0	1	0	1	82	58	91	84	21	15	8
0	1	1	0	90	83	92	85	30	6	7
0	1	1	1	86	75	90	83	27	9	9
1	0	0	0	89	61	100	92	22	14	0
1	0	0	1	90	64	100	92	23	13	0
1	0	1	0	94	81	99	91	29	7	1
1	0	1	1	91	78	96	88	28	8	4
1	1	0	0	91	67	100	92	24	12	0
1	1	0	1	91	72	99	91	26	10	1
1	1	1	0	91	81	96	88	29	7	4
1	1	1	1	91	81	95	87	29	7	5

[a]The value of '0' means that the feature does not occur, '1' that it occurs in calculations

5.3 Discriminant Analysis

Discriminant analysis [32–38] feasible in Matlab is associated with the function classify. It enabled to implement one possible type of discriminant function— quadratic (fits multivariate normal densities with covariance estimates stratified by group) in the function GUI_hyperspectral_class_disc. Besides the above type, it is possible to use the following discriminant functions [35–37]:

- linear—fits a multivariate normal density to each group,
- diaglinear—with a diagonal covariance matrix estimate.
- diagquadratic—with a diagonal covariance matrix estimate.
- mahalanobis—uses Mahalanobis distances with stratified covariance estimates.

Implementation of a discriminant function in the function GUI_hyperspec-tral_class_disc is as follows:

```
...
grpname = classify(measT,meas,species','quadratic');
TP=sum( strcmp(grpname,'Yes').* strcmp(species','Yes')
); %
TN=sum( strcmp(grpname,'No') .* strcmp(species','No')
); %
FN=sum( strcmp(grpname,'No') .* strcmp(species','Yes')
); %
FP=sum( strcmp(grpname,'Yes').* strcmp(species','No')
); %
ACC= round((TP+TN)/(FN+FP+TN+TP).*100);
TPR= round(TP/(TP+FN).*100);
SPC= round(TN/(TN+FP).*100);
...
```

The above excerpt provides the results presented in Fig. 5.4.

Similarly to the previously discussed classifiers, in Fig. 5.4 negative and positive cases (wavelengths) are marked in green and red and the classification function in blue: in Fig. 5.4a for features: intensity ($L_{INT}(i)$), homogeneity ($L_{HOM}(i)$) and energy ($L_{ENE}(i)$); in Fig. 5.4b for features: contrast ($L_{CON}(i)$), homogeneity ($L_{HOM}(i)$) and energy ($L_{ENE}(i)$). For these and other combinations of features, the numerical results of *ACC, TPR, SPC, TN, TP, FN, FP* are shown in Table 5.3.

In Table 5.3, there is only one case when *ACC* = 95%. This is the accuracy value for the combination of features *INT* and *CON*. The minimum value of accuracy is 65% and occurs for a single feature *HOM*.

As mentioned above, discriminant analysis enables to use different types of discriminant function. Figure 5.5 and Table 5.4 show the results obtained for three features (homogeneity, intensity and energy) for various types of discriminant analysis: 'linear', 'diaglinear', 'diagquadratic' and 'mahalanobis'.

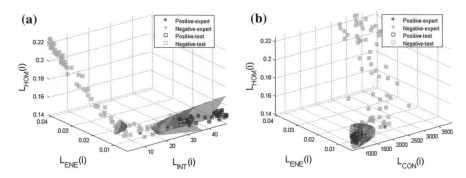

Fig. 5.4 Results of classification, discriminant analysis—'quadratic'. Negative and positive cases (wavelengths) are marked in *green* and *red* and the classification function in blue: **a** for features: intensity ($L_{INT}(i)$), homogeneity ($L_{HOM}(i)$) and energy ($L_{ENE}(i)$); **b** for features: contrast ($L_{CON}(i)$), homogeneity ($L_{HOM}(i)$) and energy ($L_{ENE}(i)$)

Table 5.3 Results of *TN, TP, FN, FP* as well as *ACC, TPR, SPC* (expressed as a percentage) for discriminant analysis for different combinations of features—on/off position of checkbox objects (*INT, ENE, VAR, HOM*)[a]

INT	CON	ENE	HOM	ACC	TPR	SPC	TN	TP	FN	FP
0	0	0	1	65	50	71	65	18	18	27
0	0	1	0	91	92	90	83	33	3	9
0	0	1	1	84	75	87	80	27	9	12
0	1	0	0	88	83	90	83	30	6	9
0	1	0	1	84	75	88	81	27	9	11
0	1	1	0	87	92	85	78	33	3	14
0	1	1	1	88	92	86	79	33	3	13
1	0	0	0	92	72	100	92	26	10	0
1	0	0	1	91	75	97	89	27	9	3
1	0	1	0	94	94	93	86	34	2	6
1	0	1	1	94	94	93	86	34	2	6
1	1	0	0	95	86	98	90	31	5	2
1	1	0	1	94	94	93	86	34	2	6
1	1	1	0	90	94	88	81	34	2	11
1	1	1	1	90	97	87	80	35	1	12

[a]The value of '0' means that the feature does not occur, '1' that it occurs in calculations

Different results, presented in Table 5.4, are obtained depending on the selected type of discriminant analysis.

The best results (Table 5.4) are for 'mahalanobis' type of discriminant analysis, i.e. *ACC* = 97%. The worst results are for 'diagquadratic' type, i.e. *ACC* = 92%. The differences arise directly from the type of analysis and the distribution of values of individual features.

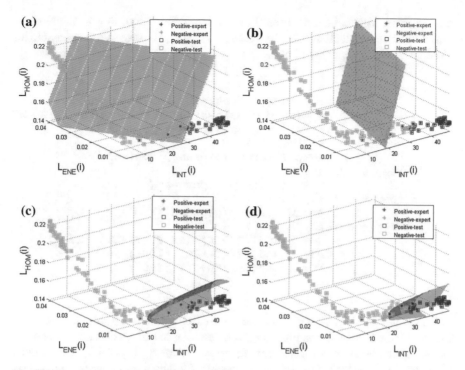

Fig. 5.5 Results of classification for three features—homogeneity $L_{HOM}(i)$), intensity ($L_{INT}(i)$) and energy ($L_{ENE}(i)$) for different types of discriminant analysis: **a** 'linear'; **b** 'diaglinear'; **c** 'diagquadratic'; **d** 'mahalanobis'. Negative and positive cases (wavelengths) are marked in *green* and *red* and the classification function in *blue*

Table 5.4 Results of *TN, TP, FN, FP* as well as *ACC, TPR, SPC* (expressed as a percentage) for different types of discriminant analysis and the features *INT, ENE* and *HOM*

Type	ACC	TPR	SPC	TN	TP	FN	FP
Linear	93	75	100	92	27	9	0
Diaglinear	94	92	95	87	33	3	5
Quadratic	94	94	93	86	34	2	6
Diagquadratic	92	86	95	87	31	5	5
Mahalanobis	97	92	99	91	33	3	1

5.4   Support Vector Machine

Support vector machine has been one of the most popular classifiers in recent years [38–51]. It allows for the appointment of a hyperplane that enables to separate two classes [41, 42, 44] with the greatest possible margin [45–48]. The implementation of the SVM classifier was carried out in the function GUI_hyperspectral_ class_svm which, in turn, uses the function svmtrain. A fragment of the source code of the function GUI_hyperspectral_class_svm responsible for SVM classification is shown below:

```
...
                    svmStruct = svmtrain(meas,species');
                    grpname = svmclassify(svmStruct,measT);
                    TP=sum( strcmp(grpname,'Yes').*
strcmp(species','Yes') ); %
                    TN=sum( strcmp(grpname,'No') .*
strcmp(species','No') ); %
                    FN=sum( strcmp(grpname,'No') .*
strcmp(species','Yes') ); %
                    FP=sum( strcmp(grpname,'Yes').*
strcmp(species','No') ); %
                    ACC= round((TP+TN)/(FN+FP+TN+TP).*100);
                    TPR= round(TP/(TP+FN).*100);
                    SPC= round(TN/(TN+FP).*100);
...
```

The results of SVM classification are shown in Fig. 5.6 and Table 5.5. Negative and positive cases (wavelengths) (Fig. 5.6) are marked in green and red and the classification function in blue for features: intensity ($L_{INT}(i)$), homogeneity ($L_{HOM}(i)$) and energy ($L_{ENE}(i)$)—Fig. 5.6a); for features: contrast ($L_{CON}(i)$), homogeneity ($L_{HOM}(i)$) and energy ($L_{ENE}(i)$)—Fig. 5.6b).

Numerical results of individual combinations of features in the training and test vectors are shown in Table 5.5.

The greatest values of $ACC = 91\%$ were obtained for a few combinations of features ENE, ENE and HOM, INT and HOM, INT and ENE and HOM, INT and CON and HOM, INT and CON and ENE and HOM. In almost each of these

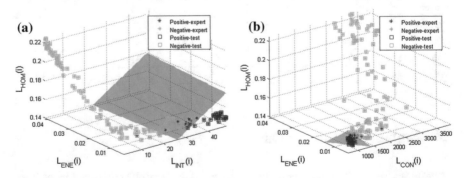

Fig. 5.6 Results of SVM classification. Negative and positive cases (wavelengths) are marked in *green* and *red* and the classification function in *blue*: **a** for features: intensity ($L_{INT}(i)$), homogeneity ($L_{HOM}(i)$) and energy ($L_{ENE}(i)$); **b** for features: contrast ($L_{CON}(i)$), homogeneity ($L_{HOM}(i)$) and energy ($L_{ENE}(i)$)

Table 5.5 Results of *TN*, *TP*, *FN*, *FP* as well as *ACC*, *TPR*, *SPC* (expressed as a percentage) for SVM for different combinations of features—on/off position of checkbox objects *(INT, ENE, VAR, HOM)*[a]

INT	CON	ENE	HOM	ACC	TPR	SPC	TN	TP	FN	FP
0	0	0	1	72	0	100	92	0	36	0
0	0	1	0	91	89	91	84	32	4	8
0	0	1	1	91	89	91	84	32	4	8
0	1	0	0	84	50	98	90	18	18	2
0	1	0	1	88	81	91	84	29	7	8
0	1	1	0	87	53	100	92	19	17	0
0	1	1	1	87	69	93	86	25	11	6
1	0	0	0	88	58	100	92	21	15	0
1	0	0	1	91	69	100	92	25	11	0
1	0	1	0	88	58	100	92	21	15	0
1	0	1	1	91	69	100	92	25	11	0
1	1	0	0	89	61	100	92	22	14	0
1	1	0	1	91	69	100	92	25	11	0
1	1	1	0	89	61	100	92	22	14	0
1	1	1	1	91	69	100	92	25	11	0

[a]The value of '0' means that the feature does not occur, '1' that it occurs in calculations

combinations, there is the feature *HOM*. The feature *ENE* is noteworthy as it is able (as a single feature) to provide the best results of accuracy for the considered SVM classifier.

Summing up, the best results for the analysed case are obtained for 'maha-lanobis' type of discriminant analysis, i.e. *ACC* = 97%. The results should be treated only illustratively as they present possible problems and methods of analysis of the results obtained from the implemented classifiers.

5.5   Receiver Operating Characteristics

The receiver operating characteristics (ROC) curve is obtained on the basis of classification results. Changes in sensitivity as a function of specificity are analysed. The individual measurement points can, in the general case, be the result of a classifier operation for different types of changes. A classic example is a change in the position of the cut-off threshold during data classification. For the described types of classifiers and the presented data, the ROC curve enables to show extremely important information, which is sensitive to changing parameters. The assessment of sensitivity relates here to resizing the averaging filter h_w (from the default parameters $M_w \times N_w = 3 \times 3$ pixels), choosing the size of the *ROIc*

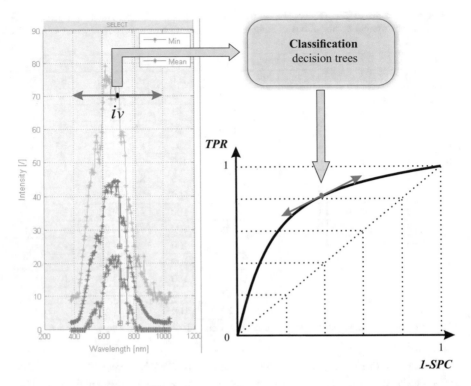

Fig. 5.7 Block diagram of calculating the values for the ROC curve and changes in the location of the *TP* area in the range of $\pm i_v$

(typically $Mc \times Nc = 40 \times 40$ pixels), choosing the size of the structural element *SE2* for conditional erosion and dilation (the default size $M_{SE2} \times N_{SE2}$), and the values of the thresholds p_{ec} and p_{dc}, classifier type (decision trees, naive Bayes classifier, SVM), choosing the threshold p_{rg}, choosing True and False areas (Fig. 4.8). The potential impact of the settings (selection) of the above variables on the results obtained must be verified in practice. The impact of changes in the last parameter—manual selection of True and False areas—has been further described in the monograph (Fig. 4.8). Figure 5.7 shows the idea of measuring the ROC curve.

A change in the range of $\pm i_v$ (Fig. 5.7) of the location of the *TP* area will affect the division into TP and TN of the training vector, a different structure of the decision tree and thus different values of *SPC* and *TPR* representing a point on the ROC plot. The source code responsible for the calculation of the various values needed to plot the ROC curve is in the function GUI_hyperspectral_class. It has been deliberately marked (symbol '%') as a comment to encourage, at this point, the readers to introduce their own element (e.g. a button) on the menu

Fig. 5.8 ROC curve for
changes in the location of the
TP area in the range of $\pm i_v$ for
$i_v = 30$

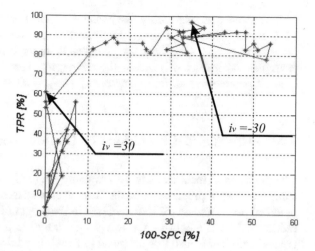

that would run the ROC analysis for changes in the range of $\pm i_v$. A fragment
of the source code responsible for changes in the range of $\pm i_v$ for $i_v = 30$ is as
follows:

```
ROC_=[];
TRR_=TRR;
for iv=1:30 % left
         TRR_=[TRR_(2:end);TRR_(1)];

[TP,TN,FP,FN,ACC,TPR,SPC]=GUI_hyperspectral_class_dec_
tree(TRR_,meas,measT,nam);
         ROC_=[ROC_;[TPR, 100-SPC]];
     end
     TRR_=TRR; % right
     for iv=1:30
         TRR_=[TRR_(end);TRR_(1:(end-1))];

[TP,TN,FP,FN,ACC,TPR,SPC]=GUI_hyperspectral_class_dec_
tree(TRR_,meas,measT,nam);
         ROC_=[ROC_;[TPR, 100-SPC]];
     end
     figure; plot(ROC_(:,2),ROC_(:,1),'-r*'); grid
on;
     xlabel('100-SPC
[%]','FontSize',14,'FontAngle','Italic');
     ylabel('TPR
[%]','FontSize',14,'FontAngle','Italic');
```

The result is the ROC curve presented in Fig. 5.8.

The above example is only one possible application of this approach for plotting ROC curves. I encourage the reader to further test and analyse changes in the value of sensitivity and specificity for changes in other aforementioned variables, for example, the impact of resizing the averaging filter h_w from $M_w \times N_w = 3 \times 3$ (default parameters) to, for example, $M_w \times N_w = 33 \times 33$ pixels.

5.6   Pitfalls and Limitations of Classification

Classification in most cases is the crowning stage of the tedious process of image analysis. Proper preparation of the data vector(s) is extremely important from a practical point of view [52]. An increase in the length of the training vector and/or a reduction in the length of the test vector improve the results obtained, but the created classifier is also less universal [53, 54]. In addition, the pressure to improve the results obtained is high, especially if the area of the publication of results in scientific journals and (almost) the need to confirm the superiority of the developed method are taken into account. Apart from changing the length of the training and test vector, also other errors can be made during classification [52, 55, 56]. The most common errors are:

- providing the results of classification for the training vector as those for the test vector,
- reducing the length of the test vector—increasing the length of the training vector (as mentioned above),
- overfitting,
- an excessive number of features at a too small vector length,
- leakage of data between the training and test data,
- artificial reproduction of data,
- failure to provide an appropriate range of variation.

Ignoring the mathematical relations and moving on to the practical implementation, two files are taken into account: `test.mat` and `reference.mat`. These files are the result of previously conducted analysis and were previously stored on the disk. After reading them and standardizing common wavelengths, an SVM classifier will be built and tested for both the training and test data. The corresponding source code (the part concerning graphs is similar to the previously described one—in previous subchapters) is shown below:

```
pathn_='D:/k/' ;
test=load([pathn_,'_I20_L0-511_13-1-
2016_13.5.59.cubetest.mat']);
reference=load([pathn_,'_I20_L0-511_13-1-
2016_13.5.59.cubereference.mat']);
measT=[];
meas=[];
for ij=1:size(test.Wavelength_,1)
    if
sum(test.Wavelength_(ij)==reference.Wavelength_)==1
        measT=[measT;test.anal(ij,4:6)];
meas=[meas;reference.anal(test.Wavelength_(ij)==refere
nce.Wavelength_,4:6)];
    end
end
%measT=meas;
TRR=zeros([size(meas,1), 1]);
TRR(20:110)=1;
species=[];
for ijj=1:length(TRR)
    if TRR(ijj)==1
        species{ijj}='Yes';
    else
        species{ijj}='No';
    end
end
svmStruct = svmtrain(meas,species');
grpname = svmclassify(svmStruct,measT);
TP=sum( strcmp(grpname,'Yes').* strcmp(species','Yes')
);
TN=sum( strcmp(grpname,'No') .* strcmp(species','No')
);
FN=sum( strcmp(grpname,'No') .* strcmp(species','Yes')
);
FP=sum( strcmp(grpname,'Yes').* strcmp(species','No')
);
ACC= round((TP+TN)/(FN+FP+TN+TP).*100)
TPR= round(TP/(TP+FN).*100);
SPC= round(TN/(TN+FP).*100);
figure;
plot3(measT(strcmp(species','Yes'),1),measT(strcmp(spe
cies','Yes'),2),measT(strcmp(species','Yes'),3),'r*');
hold on
plot3(measT(strcmp(species','No'),1),measT(strcmp(spec
ies','No'),2),measT(strcmp(species','No'),3),'g*');
plot3(measT(strcmp(grpname,'Yes'),1),measT(strcmp(grpn
ame,'Yes'),2),measT(strcmp(grpname,'Yes'),3),'rs');
plot3(measT(strcmp(grpname,'No'),1),measT(strcmp(grpna
```

```
me,'No'),2),measT(strcmp(grpname,'No'),3),'gs'); grid
on
xlabel('feature 1','FontSize',16);
ylabel('feature 2','FontSize',16);
zlabel('feature 3','FontSize',16);
LI=100;
[x,y,z]=meshgrid( lin-
space(min(measT(:,1)),max(measT(:,1)),100) , lin-
space(min(measT(:,2)),max(measT(:,2)),100)
,linspace(min(measT(:,3)),max(measT(:,3)),100));
X = x(:); Y = y(:); Z=z(:);
[v] = svmclassify(svmStruct,[X Y Z]);
v=reshape(v,LI,LI,LI);
p1 =
patch(isosurface(x,y,z,(strcmp(v,'Yes')),0.5),'FaceCol
or',[0 0 1 ],'EdgeColor','none');
view(3); axis tight
camlight; camlight(-80,-10); lighting phong;
grid on
alpha(p1,0.3)
legend('Positive-expert','Negative-expert','Positive-
test','Negative-test')
```

The results obtained for the training and test data (see %measT = meas;) are shown in Figs. 5.9 and 5.10.

The results shown in Figs. 5.9 and 5.10 are clearly better (a change in *ACC* from 41 to 89% for the training vector). However, the classifier due to its characteristics does not fit to the data (there is no problem of overfitting).

The second discussed issue is reducing the length of the test vector. Let us assume the length u of the test vector is changed from 1 (one positive or negative case) to 100 cases (the number of positive and negative cases is random), i.e. $u \in (1, 100)$. The results obtained are shown in the graph in Fig. 5.11.

Fig. 5.9 Results of the SVM classification for exemplary features of the training data. *TP* = 85, *TN* = 24, *FN* = 6, *FP* = 7, *ACC* = 89%, *TPR* = 93%, *SPC* = 77%

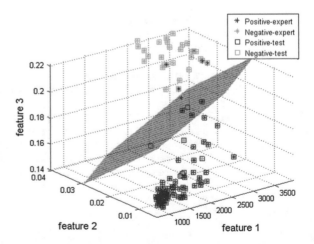

Fig. 5.10 Results of the
SVM classification for
exemplary features of the test
data. $TP = 19$, $TN = 31$,
$FN = 72$, $FP = 0$,
$ACC = 41\%$, $TPR = 21\%$,
$SPC = 100\%$

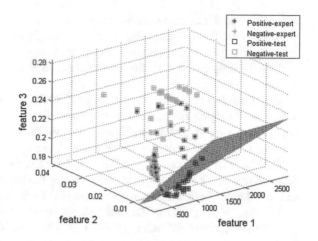

Fig. 5.11 Graph of changes
in ACC for different lengths of
the test vector

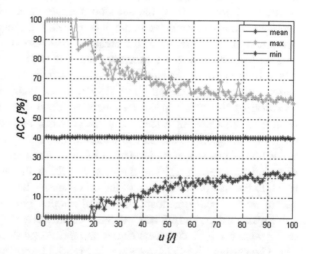

The results shown in the graph in Fig. 5.11 relate to changes in ACC for different lengths of the test vector. Each value of u is the result of 1000 random data. Accordingly, the maximum values are marked in green (Fig. 5.11), whereas the minimum ones in blue. The presented graph indicates almost complete dependence of the result (ACC) on the appropriate selection of data if there are no more than 10 of them (for the considered case). The more data are drawn, the narrower the range of variability of ACC. In an extreme case, $ACC = 40 \pm 20\%$ in the graph in Fig. 5.11. To sum up, a reduction in the length of the test vector allows for almost any change in the results of, for example, accuracy.

The third discussed issue is overfitting. Overfitting the data is typical for most classifiers. For example, this is the induction of binary decision trees without pruning. This problem is mentioned in the subchapter "Decision trees". Figure 5.2b shows a graph of dependence of cross-validation errors on the number of tree nodes. The problem of overfitting produces very good results of accuracy, sensitivity and specificity. Unfortunately, an induced decision tree (classifier) is not able to generalize data, so its practical clinical usefulness is limited. Overfitting the data applies not only to the classifier construction. It is also related to the type of data source.

The induction of the decision tree for data from a single source, one hospital and/or one imaging device, causes excessive fit to the data despite, for example, pruning the tree. A similar problem occurs in the analysis of data from a single operator (physician) operating the imaging device.

The discussed issues are well illustrated by the example of the induction of a decision tree for the training data and showing the results obtained for the training and test data of both the complete and pruned decision tree—Table 5.6.

The results presented in Table 5.6 show small differences in accuracy for the pruned trees and test and training data (5%). There are also big differences between the test and training data obtained for the complete decision tree—the difference in accuracy of 35%. Pruning the decision tree produces worse results but the created decision tree is less sensitive to the data. In addition, transparency increases and the computational complexity of the created tree decreases.

The fourth issue is an excessive number of features in relation to the vector length (number of analysed cases). To some extent this is justified. In the case of the tedious process of designing the algorithm for analysis and processing, the culmination of this work is the data vector—the vector of features. Adding a new feature is the result of a small amount of work compared to the said process of algorithm designing. Therefore, the authors of various works induce a classifier and test it for dozens and even hundreds of features which are acquired from only a few cases of data (patients). The question to which the answer will be given below refers to the maximum number of features that can be used for classification so as to obtain reliable and diagnostically useful results. For this purpose, the SVM classifier was used and a different number of features $k \in (1, 50)$ and different lengths of the vector $u \in (4, 50)$ were chosen at random (uniform distribution in the set $\{0, 1\}$). The results of ACC are shown in Fig. 5.11 and Fig. 5.12.

The source code for performing these calculations and creating the graph shown in Fig. 5.11 is as follows:

Table 5.6 Results of TN, TP, FN, FP as well as ACC, TPR, SPC (expressed as a percentage) for the complete and pruned decision tree for the training and test data

Decision tree	Data type	ACC	TPR	SPC	TN	TP	FN	FP
Complete	Training[a]	92	91	92	52	60	5	5
Complete	Test	57	26	85	15	55	42	10
Pruned	Training	73	75	71	43	46	14	19
Pruned	Test	68	79	58	45	38	12	27

[a]The lack of specificity, sensitivity and accuracy equal to 100% for the complete decision tree and the test data is due to 10-fold cross-validation of data which is determined by default

```
res=[]; h = waitbar(0,'Please wait...');
for u=4:50
    TRR=rand([u 1])<0.5;
    species=[];
    for ijj=1:length(TRR)
        if TRR(ijj)==1
            species{ijj}='Yes';
        else
            species{ijj}='No';
        end
    end
    for k=1:50
        meas=rand([u k]);
        svmStruct = svmtrain(meas,species');
        grpname = svmclassify(svmStruct,meas);
        TP=sum( strcmp(grpname,'Yes').*
strcmp(species','Yes') );
        TN=sum( strcmp(grpname,'No') .*
strcmp(species','No') );
        FN=sum( strcmp(grpname,'No') .*
strcmp(species','Yes') );
        FP=sum( strcmp(grpname,'Yes').*
strcmp(species','No') );
        ACC= round((TP+TN)/(FN+FP+TN+TP).*100);
        res=[res;[u,k,ACC]];
    end
    waitbar(u/100,h)
end
close(h)
figure; plot3(res(:,1),res(:,2),res(:,3),'r*'); hold
on; grid on;
xlabel('u [/]','FontSize',14,'FontAngle','Italic')
ylabel('k [/]','FontSize',14,'FontAngle','Italic')
zlabel('ACC [%]','FontSize',14,'FontAngle','Italic')
```

The result of changes in *ACC* as a function of changes in the number of features and vector length shown in Fig. 5.11 is of great practical importance. It enables to determine the minimum u/k ratio which provides diagnostically useful results. Figure 5.13 shows the dependence of ACC as a function of u/k which shows that for $u/k = 10$ and less, the results exceed the value of 50% of accuracy. This means that the classification accuracy of the classifier, regardless of the data (they may be even random), is well above 50%, and for $u/k = 5$ and less accuracy is approximately 100%. Therefore, the practical utility of such a classifier is questionable. It is therefore necessary to provide in each case at least several-fold increase in the training vector length in relation to the number of features.

The fifth problem is the data leakage between the training and test data. The leakage is further understood as the overlap of data from the training and test vectors. If we assume that *s* will mean the percentage overlap of the two data

Fig. 5.12 Graph of changes
in *ACC* for different lengths of
the test vector *u* and a
different number of features *k*

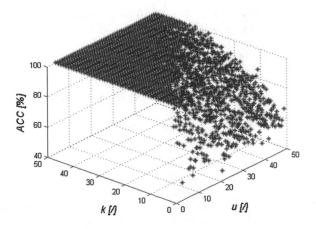

vectors, the result of accuracy (*ACC*) for different values of $s \in (0, 100)$ will run for the SVM classifier in accordance with the graph shown in Fig. 5.14.

According to the graph shown in Fig. 5.14 and as expected, the larger the percentage share of the test vector in the training vector, the better the results obtained. For example, for a few per cent (from 0 to about 20) of common data, the value of *ACC* does not change. For *s* ranging from 40 to 85%, the value of *ACC* increased by 9%. It should be noted here that data leakage is mainly associated with the wrong (intended or unintended) implementation of the classifier.

The last mentioned problems, i.e. artificial duplication of data and failure to provide an adequate range of variability of data, have already been partially discussed in the previous problems.

In the presented application related to hyperspectral images, the number of features is disproportionately smaller than the length of the data vector ($i = 128$ for 4 features). Lack of data leakage ensures proper implementation of the transformations discussed in earlier chapters. Only deliberate action, such as reducing the

Fig. 5.13 Graph of changes
in *ACC* for different values of
the ratio of the test vector
length *u* to the number of
features *k*

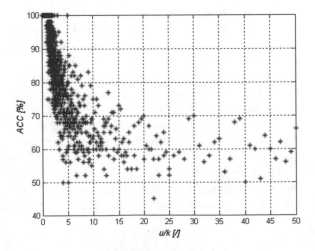

Fig. 5.14 Graph of changes
in *ACC* for different *s* degrees
of overlap of the test vector
and the training vector

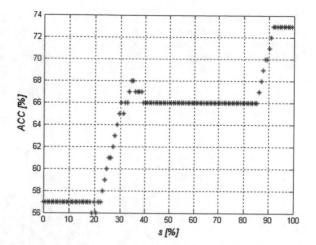

training vector length to several 2D images can cause the discussed problems. At this point, I encourage the reader to create appropriate warnings for the application user about the occurrence of one of the discussed problems, for example using the function warndlg('Data leakage','!! Warning !!').

The source codes of all the discussed problems have been saved in separate *m-files* in the materials attached to this monograph, namely Class_test, Class_test2, Class_test3, Class_test4 and Class_test5.

5.7   Blok Diagram of the Discussed Transformations

The block diagram of the discussed issues is presented in Fig. 5.15.

The block diagram presented in Fig. 5.15 concerns the algorithm part responsible for the selection of a classifier. Depending on the operator's individual choice, it is possible to analyse in the proposed application the results obtained for the following classifiers: decision trees, naive Bayes classifier, discriminant analysis and support vector machine. In Matlab in Statistics Toolbox, implementation of other types of classifications, e.g., k-means, is also possible. I encourage the readers at this point to perform their own implementation of the above functions for one of the possible definitions of distance, i.e.: 'sqEuclidean' (squared euclidean distance); 'cityblock' (sum of absolute differences); 'cosine' (one minus the cosine of the included angle between points); 'correlation' (one minus the sample correlation between points); 'Hamming'—(percentage of bits that differ).

Fig. 5.15 Block diagram of
the algorithm part responsible
for the selection of a classifier
and for the ROC curves

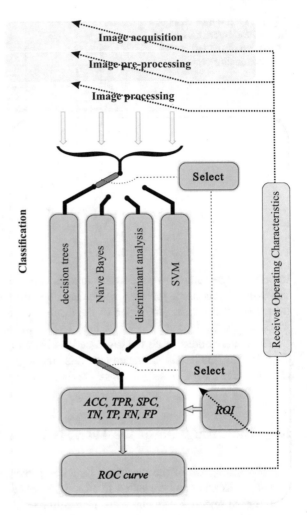

References

1. Ye F, Chen ZH, Chen J, Liu F, Zhang Y, Fan QY, Wang L Chi-squared Automatic Interaction Detection Decision Tree Analysis of Risk Factors for Infant Anemia in Beijing, China. Chin Med J (Engl). 2016 20th May;129(10):1193–1199. doi:10.4103/0366-6999.181955.
2. Heikkilä P, Forma L, Korppi M. High-flow oxygen therapy is more cost-effective for bronchiolitis than standard treatment-a decision-tree analysis. Pediatr Pulmonol. 2016 May 5
3. Kadi I, Idri A. Cardiovascular Dysautonomias Diagnosis Using Crisp and Fuzzy Decision Tree: A Comparative Study. Stud Health Technol Inform. 2016;223:1–8.
4. Kraszewska-Głomba B, Szymańska-Toczek Z, Szenborn L. Procalcitonin and C-reactive protein-based decision tree model for distinguishing PFAPA flares from acute infections. Bosn J Basic Med Sci. 2016 Mar 10;16(2):157–61. doi:10.17305/bjbms.2016.974.

5. Fernández L, Mediano P, García R, Rodríguez JM, Marín M. Risk Factors Predicting Infectious Lactational Mastitis: Decision Tree Approach versus Logistic Regression Analysis. Matern Child Health J. 2016 Apr 11. [Epub ahead of print]

6. Garcia RJ, von Winterfeldt D. Defender-Attacker Decision Tree Analysis to Combat Terrorism. Risk Anal. 2016 Apr 1. doi:10.1111/risa.12574. [Epub ahead of print]

7. Bamber JH, Evans SA. The value of decision tree analysis in planning anaesthetic care in obstetrics. Int J Obstet Anesth. 2016 Feb 27. pii: S0959-289X(16)00036-4. doi:10.1016/j.ijoa. 2016.02.007. [Epub ahead of print] Review.

8. Leach HJ, O'Connor DP, Simpson RJ, Rifai HS, Mama SK, Lee RE. An exploratory decision tree analysis to predict cardiovascular disease risk in African American women. Health Psychol. 2016 Apr;35(4):397–402. doi:10.1037/hea0000267.

9. Wylie CE, Shaw DJ, Verheyen KL, Newton JR. Decision-tree analysis of clinical data to aid diagnostic reasoning for equine laminitis: a cross-sectional study. Vet Rec. 2016 Apr 23;178 (17):420. doi:10.1136/vr.103588. Epub 2016 Mar 11.

10. Oksel C, Winkler DA, Ma CY, Wilkins T, Wang XZ. Accurate and interpretable nanoSAR models from genetic programming-based decision tree construction approaches. Nanotoxicology. 2016 Apr 6:1–12. [Epub ahead of print]

11. Montorsi F, Oelke M, Henneges C, Brock G, Salonia A, d'Anzeo G, Rossi A, Mulhall JP, Büttner H. Exploratory Decision-Tree Modeling of Data from the Randomized REACTT Trial of Tadalafil Versus Placebo to Predict Recovery of Erectile Function After Bilateral Nerve-Sparing Radical Prostatectomy. Eur Urol. 2016 Mar 3. pii: S0302-2838(16)00214-1. doi:10.1016/j.eururo.2016.02.036. [Epub ahead of print]

12. Baneshi MR, Haghdoost AA, Zolala F, Nakhaee N, Jalali M, Tabrizi R, Akbari M. Can Religious Beliefs be a Protective Factor for Suicidal Behavior? A Decision Tree Analysis in a Mid-Sized City in Iran, 2013. J Relig Health. 2016 Feb 29. [Epub ahead of print]

13. Medeiros LB, Trigueiro DR, Silva DM, Nascimento JA, Monroe AA, Nogueira JA, Leadebal OD. Integration of health services in the care of people living with aids: an approach using a decision tree Cien Saude Colet. 2016 Feb;21(2):543–552. English, Portuguese.

14. Hashem S, Esmat G, Elakel W, Habashy S, Abdel Raouf S, Darweesh S, Soliman M, Elhefnawi M, El-Adawy M, ElHefnawi M. Accurate Prediction of Advanced Liver Fibrosis Using the Decision Tree Learning Algorithm in Chronic Hepatitis C Egyptian Patients. Gastroenterol Res Pract. 2016;2016:2636390. doi:10.1155/2016/2636390. Epub 2016 Jan 6.

15. Collet JF, Lacave R, Hugonin S, Poulot V, Tassart M, Fajac A. BRAF V600E detection in cytological thyroid samples: A key component of the decision tree for surgical treatment of papillary thyroid carcinoma. Head Neck. 2016 Feb 8. doi:10.1002/hed.24393. [Epub ahead of print]

16. Kang Y, McHugh MD, Chittams J, Bowles KH. Utilizing Home Healthcare Electronic Health Records for Telehomecare Patients With Heart Failure: A Decision Tree Approach to Detect Associations With Rehospitalizations. Comput Inform Nurs. 2016 Apr;34(4):175–82. doi:10. 1097/CIN.0000000000000223.

17. Owen EB, Woods CR, O'Flynn JA, Boone MC, Calhoun AW, Montgomery VL. A Bedside Decision Tree for Use of Saline With Endotracheal Tube Suctioning in Children. Crit Care Nurse. 2016 Feb;36(1):e1–e10. doi:10.4037/ccn2016358.

18. Asafu-Adjei JK, Betensky RA.A Pairwise Naïve Bayes Approach to Bayesian Classification. Intern J Reference Recognit Artif Intell. 2015 Oct 1;29(7). pii: 1550023.

19. Chen C, Zhang G, Yang J, Milton JC, Alcántara AD. An explanatory analysis of driver injury severity in rear-end crashes using a decision table/Naïve Bayes (DTNB) hybrid classifier. Accid Anal Prev. 2016 May;90:95–107.

20. Geng H, Lu T, Lin X, Liu Y, Yan F. Prediction of Protein-Protein Interaction Sites Based on Naive Bayes Classifier. Biochem Res Int. 2015;2015:978193.

21. Miasnikof P, Giannakeas V, Gomes M, Aleksandrowicz L, Shestopaloff AY, Alam D, Tollman S, Samarikhalaj A, Jha P. Naive Bayes classifiers for verbal autopsies: comparison to physician-based classification for 21,000 child and adult deaths. BMC Med. 2015 Nov 25;13:286.

22. Griffis JC, Allendorfer JB, Szaflarski JP. Voxel-based Gaussian naïve Bayes classification of ischemic stroke lesions in individual T1-weighted MRI scans. J Neurosci Methods. 2016 Jan 15;257:97–108.

23. Wang M, Zuo W, Wang Y. A Multilayer Naïve Bayes Model for Analyzing User's Retweeting Sentiment Tendency. Comput Intell Neurosci. 2015;2015:510281.

24. Marucci-Wellman HR, Lehto MR, Corns HL.A practical tool for public health surveillance: Semi-automated coding of short injury narratives from large administrative databases using Naïve Bayes algorithms. Accid Anal Prev. 2015 Nov;84:165–76. doi:10.1016/j.aap.2015.06. 014. Epub 2015 Sep 26.

25. Carvajal G, Roser DJ, Sisson SA, Keegan A, Khan SJ. Modelling pathogen log10 reduction values achieved by activated sludge treatment using naïve and semi naïve Bayes network models. Water Res. 2015 Nov 15;85:304–15. doi:10.1016/j.watres.2015.08.035. Epub 2015 Aug 21.

26. Dou Y, Guo X, Yuan L, Holding DR, Zhang C. Differential Expression Analysis in RNA-Seq by a Naive Bayes Classifier with Local Normalization. Biomed Res Int. 2015;2015:789516.

27. Pogodin PV, Lagunin AA, Filimonov DA, Poroikov VV. PASS Targets: Ligand-based multi-target computational system based on a public data and naïve Bayes approach. SAR QSAR Environ Res. 2015;26(10):783–93.

28. Waleska Simões P, Mazzuchello LL, Toniazzo de Abreu LL, Garcia D, dos Passos MG, Venson R, Bisognin Ceretta L, Veiga Silva AC, da Rosa MI, Martins PJ. A Comparative Study of Bayes Net, Naive Bayes and Averaged One-Dependence Estimators for Osteoporosis Analysis. Stud Health Technol Inform. 2015;216:1075.

29. Minnier J, Yuan M, Liu JS, Cai T.Risk Classification with an Adaptive Naive Bayes Kernel Machine Model. J Am Stat Assoc. 2015 Apr 22;110(509):393–404.

30. Zhang H, Yu P, Zhang TG, Kang YL, Zhao X, Li YY, He JH, Zhang J. In silico prediction of drug-induced myelotoxicity by using Naïve Bayes method. Mol Divers. 2015 Nov;19(4): 945–53.

31. Prinyakupt J, Pluempitiwiriyawej C. Segmentation of white blood cells and comparison of cell morphology by linear and naïve Bayes classifiers. Biomed Eng Online. 2015 Jun 30;14:63. doi:10.1186/s12938-015-0037-1.

32. Close ME, Abraham P, Humphries B, Lilburne L, Cuthill T, Wilson S. Predicting groundwater redox status on a regional scale using linear discriminant analysis. J Contam Hydrol. 2016 Apr 29;191:19–32.

33. Wu D, Fu X, Wen Y, Liu B, Deng Z, Dai L, Tan D. High-resolution melting combines with Bayes discriminant analysis: a novel hepatitis C virus genotyping method. Clin Exp Med. 2016 May 13.

34. McDonald LS, Panozzo JF, Salisbury PA, Ford R. Discriminant Analysis of Defective and Non-Defective Field Pea (Pisum sativum L.) into Broad Market Grades Based on Digital Image Features. PLoS One. 2016 May 13;11(5):e0155523.

35. Han B, Peng H, Yan H. Identification of Medicinal Mugua Origin by Near Infrared Spectroscopy Combined with Partial Least-squares Discriminant Analysis. Pharmacogn Mag. 2016 Apr-Jun;12(46):93–7.

36. Mandelkow H, de Zwart JA, Duyn JH. Linear Discriminant Analysis Achieves High Classification Accuracy for the BOLD fMRI Response to Naturalistic Movie Stimuli. Front Hum Neurosci. 2016 Mar 31;10:128.

37. Amores-Ampuero A, Alemán I. Comparison of cranial sex determination by discriminant analysis and logistic regression. Anthropol Anz. 2016 Apr 5:1–8.

38. Abbruzzo A, Tamburo E, Varrica D, Dongarrà G, Mineo A. Penalized linear discriminant analysis and Discrete AdaBoost to distinguish human hair metal profiles: The case of adolescents residing near Mt. Etna. Chemosphere. 2016 Jun;153:100–6.

39. Utkin LV, Chekh AI, Zhuk YA. Binary classification SVM-based algorithms with interval-valued training data using triangular and Epanechnikov kernels. Neural Netw. 2016 Apr 27;80:53–66.

40. Ghandi M, Mohammad-Noori M, Ghareghani N, Lee D, Garraway L, Beer MA. gkmSVM: an R package for gapped-kmer SVM. Bioinformatics. 2016 Apr 19. pii: btw203.
41. Lee D. LS-GKM: a new gkm-SVM for large-scale datasets. Bioinformatics. 2016 Mar 15. pii: btw142.
42. Wang X, Du H, Tan JOnline Fault Diagnosis for Biochemical Process Based on FCM and SVM. Interdiscip Sci. 2016 Apr 29.
43. Wang MY, Li P, Qiao PL. The Virtual Screening of the Drug Protein with a Few Crystal Structures Based on the Adaboost-SVM. Comput Math Methods Med. 2016;2016:4809831.
44. Sun H, Pan P, Tian S, Xu L, Kong X, Li Y, Dan Li, Hou T. Constructing and Validating High-Performance MIEC-SVM Models in Virtual Screening for Kinases: A Better Way for Actives Discovery. Sci Rep. 2016 Apr 22;6:24817.
45. Astorino A, Fuduli A. The Proximal Trajectory Algorithm in SVM Cross Validation. IEEE Trans Neural Netw Learn Syst. 2016 May;27(5):966–77.
46. Kong Y, Qu D, Chen X, Gong YN, Yan A. Self-Organizing Map (SOM) and Support Vector Machine (SVM) Models for the Prediction of Human Epidermal Growth Factor Receptor (EGFR/ ErbB-1) Inhibitors. Comb Chem High Throughput Screen. 2016;19(5):400–11.
47. Huang X, Shi L, Suykens JA. Solution Path for Pin-SVM Classifiers With Positive and Negative τ Values. IEEE Trans Neural Netw Learn Syst. 2016 Apr 8.
48. Bogaarts JG, Gommer ED, Hilkman DM, van Kranen-Mastenbroek VH, Reulen JP. Optimal training dataset composition for SVM-based, age-independent, automated epileptic seizure detection. Med Biol Eng Comput. 2016 Mar 31.
49. Peker M. A decision support system to improve medical diagnosis using a combination of k-medoids clustering based attribute weighting and SVM. J Med Syst. 2016 May;40(5):116.
50. Kieslich CA, Smadbeck J, Khoury GA, Floudas CA. conSSert: Consensus SVM Model for Accurate Prediction of Ordered Secondary Structure. J Chem Inf Model. 2016 Mar 28;56 (3):455–61.
51. Ju Z, Cao JZ, Gu H. Predicting lysine phosphoglycerylation with fuzzy SVM by incorporating k-spaced amino acid pairs into Chou's general PseAAC. J Theor Biol. 2016 May 21;397: 145–50.
52. Foster, K.R., Koprowski, R., Skufca, J.D.: Machine learning, medical diagnosis, and biomedical engineering research—commentary. Biomed. Eng. Online 13, 94 (2014).
53. Smialowski P, Frishman D, Kramer S. Pitfalls of supervised feature selection. Bioinformatics. 2010;26(3):440–443.
54. Ennett CM, Frize M. Selective Sampling to Overcome Skewed a priori Probabilities. Proceed AMIA Symposium. 2000. pp. 225–229
55. Steyerberg EW, Bleeker SE, Moll HA, Grobbee DE, Moons KG. Internal and external validation of predictive models: a simulation study of bias and precision in small samples. J Clin Epidemiol. 2003;56(5):441–447
56. Cyran KA, Kawulok J, Kawulok M, Stawarz M, Michalak M, Pietrowska M, Polańska J. Support Vector Machines in Biomedical and Biometrical Applications. In Emerging Paradigms in Machine Learning. Springer Berlin Heidelberg. 2013;13:379–417.

Chapter 6
Sensitivity to Parameter Changes

In every algorithm and software, especially those designed for the needs of medicine, it is important to assess the algorithm sensitivity to parameter changes [1]. This evaluation should be a standard item for each algorithm. Unfortunately, this is rarely encountered in practice. The authors of the new software solutions do not mention these parameters in fear of both lack of interest of buyers of the created software and the possibility of rejection of the scientific article for that reason. Sensitivity to parameter changes of any algorithm is usually strongly related to its internal structure (e.g. setting the parameters of its operation automatically) and the test method (selection of a method for changing parameters) [2, 3]. It should be emphasized here that each algorithm allows for errors at the level of 100% in extreme cases of its application [4, 5]. Therefore, it is very important to link the range of variability of parameters with the error value.

In the case of medical hyperspectral imaging, the issue of sensitivity to parameter changes is not easier. In practical terms, there are numerous different combinations of measured features and parameter changes. It is difficult to separate those combinations that are not only the most interesting but also the most diagnostically important. Certainly the most interesting element is the analysis of the sensitivity of patient positioning and the whole image acquisition on the classification results. This area, however, due to its specificity (very high dependence on the affected place and the type and severity of the disease), is left to the reader. Below there is a narrower analysis of the algorithm sensitivity to parameter

© Springer International Publishing AG 2017
R. Koprowski, *Processing of Hyperspectral Medical Images*,
Studies in Computational Intelligence 682,
DOI 10.1007/978-3-319-50490-2_6

changes. The selected parameter is the mean brightness of the manually selected *ROI*. The size of the *ROI* and its position relative to the original one (specified by the operator) will be changed.

The evaluation of the algorithm sensitivity in the evaluation of the mean brightness value for each i frame of the image $L_{GRAY}(m, n, i)$ was performed for repositioning the *ROI*, resizing the *ROI* and its rotation around its axis. The results obtained are presented in the following subchapters. The evaluation criterion J_M in each case is defined as:

$$J_M(i) = \frac{L_{MROIT}(i) - L_{MROIP}(i)}{1} \cdot 100\% \tag{6.1}$$

where

$L_{MROIT}(i)$ and $L_{MROIP}(i)$ are the mean brightness values for subsequent *ROIs*. The value of '1' results from the adopted range of the brightness level (from 0 to 1 —variable type `double`).

For example $L_{MROIT}(i)$ is equal to:

$$L_{MROIT}(i) = \frac{1}{M_{ROI} \times N_{ROI}} \sum_{m,n \in ROI} L_{GRAY}(m, n, i) \tag{6.2}$$

where M_{ROI} and N_{ROI} are the number of rows and columns of the *ROI*.

6.1 Respositioning the ROI

Repositioning the ROI involves changing its position in the row axis by Δm and in the column axis by Δn. The position of the *ROI*, in accordance with the operator's selection, shown in Fig. 4.11 was adopted by default. Its position was changed in the range $\Delta m = \pm 10$ pixels and $\Delta n = \pm 10$ pixels. The resolution of the *ROI* was $M_{ROI} \times N_{ROI} = 100 \times 100$ pixels. The results obtained are shown in Figs. 6.1 and 6.2.

The presented graphs of sensitivity to repositioning the *ROI* show that the brightness changes are smaller than $\pm 2\%$. The source code providing the graph shown in Fig. 6.1 is as follows:

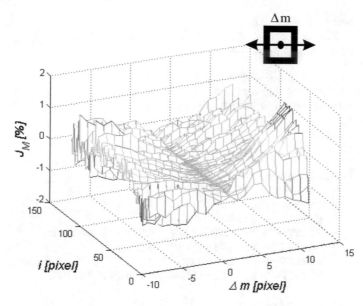

Fig. 6.1 Graph of changes in J_M for different values of Δm and subsequent i images

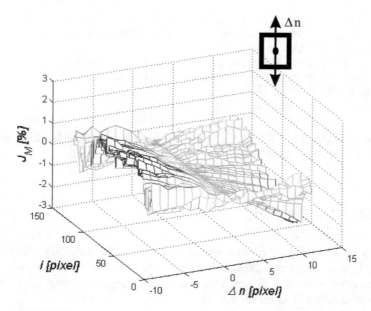

Fig. 6.2 Graph of changes in J_M for different values of Δn and subsequent i images

```
L1=load(['D:/k/_I20_L0-511_13-1-
2016_13.5.59.cube',mat2str(80),'.mat']);
Lgrayi=mat2gray(L1.L1);
figure;
[X,Y,I2,RECTP] = IMCROP(Lgrayi);
Lgrayi=IMCROP(Lgrayi,RECTP);
hObj=waitbar(0,'Please wait...');
JM=[];
for i=1:128
    L1=load(['D:/k/_I20_L0-511_13-1-
2016_13.5.59.cube',mat2str(i),'.mat']);
    Lgrayi=mat2gray(L1.L1);
    LgrayiP=IMCROP(Lgrayi,RECTP);
    LMROIP=mean(LgrayiP(:));
    for deltam=-10:10
        RECTT=RECTP; RECTT(2)=RECTT(2)+deltam;
        LgrayiT=IMCROP(Lgrayi,RECTT);
        LMROIT=mean(LgrayiT(:));
        JM(i,deltam+11)=(LMROIT-LMROIP)*100;
    end
    waitbar(i/128)
end
close(hObj)
[i,deltam]=meshgrid((1:size(JM,2))-10,1:size(JM,1));
figure
mesh(i,deltam,JM); grid on; hold on
ylabel('i [pixel]','FontSize',14,'FontAngle','Italic')
xlabel('\Delta m
[pixel]','FontSize',14,'FontAngle','Italic')
zlabel('J_M [%]','FontSize',14,'FontAngle','Italic')
view(-25,32)
```

Similar results (Figs. 6.1 and 6.2) are obtained for resizing the *ROI*, which is presented in the next subchapter.

6.2 Resizing the ROI

The impact of resizing the *ROI* (as specified above) on the percentage change in the mean brightness was determined in the same way as in the previous subchapter. In this case, the size $M \times N$ was changed in the range $\Delta M == \pm 10$ pixels and $\Delta N == \pm 10$ pixels. The results are shown in Figs. 6.3 and 6.4.

Similarly to the results obtained in the previous subchapter, the sensitivity of the brightness change to resizing the *ROI* is less than $\pm 2\%$. The next subchapter presents the effect of rotation on the change in the mean brightness in the *ROI*.

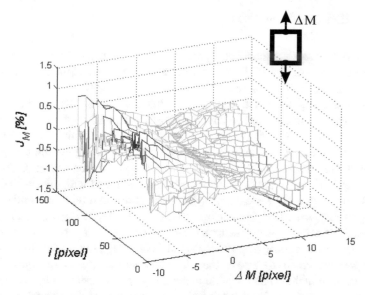

Fig. 6.3 Graph of changes in J_M for different values of ΔM and subsequent i images

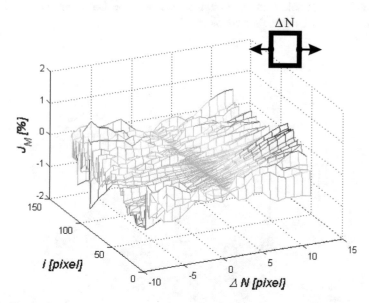

Fig. 6.4 Graph of changes in J_M for different values of ΔN and subsequent i images

6.3   Rotation of the ROI

Similarly to the previous subchapters, the algorithm sensitivity (the mean brightness value) to rotation of the *ROI* (as specified above) was verified. In this case, the rotation λ ranged from $0°$ to $360°$ (Fig. 6.5).

In this case, slightly worse results were obtained. Sensitivity to rotation of the *ROI* is the greatest in comparison with its repositioning and resizing. It is related not only to the participation of new pixels resulting from the rotation of the ROI itself but also from interpolation problems and the method of filling the missing pixels in the corners (see the function `imrotate` with the parameter 'crop'). The sensitivity values in this case are not greater than 15% compared with the absolute value. The full source code for the examples discussed above can be found in the m–files `GUI_hyperspectral_para_changes`, `GUI_hyperspectral_para_changes2`, `GUI_hyperspectral_para_changes3` and `GUI_hyperspectral_para_changes4`. Once again I encourage the readers to create their own *m-files* designed to assess the algorithm sensitivity to changes in other parameters or to include classification in the analysis. Extension of this analysis will provide a lot of useful and new information on the nature of the algorithm operation and its weaknesses. Especially the latter makes the operator more attentive to their skilful and careful selection. The analysis can also be based on the ROC curves presented in one of the earlier chapters.

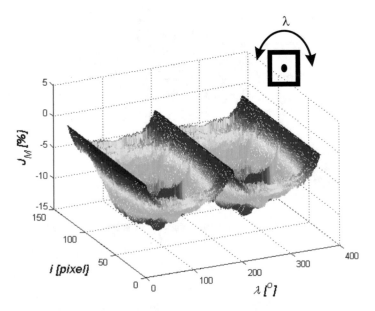

Fig. 6.5 Graph of changes in J_M for different values of λ and subsequent i images

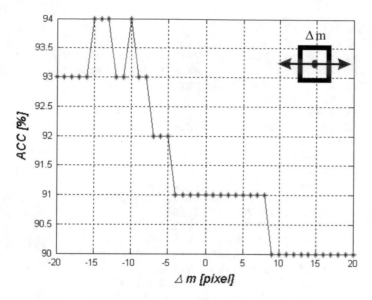

Fig. 6.6 Graph of changes in *ACC* for different values of *Δm*

6.4   The Other Parameters

The analysis of the algorithm sensitivity to parameter changes is a broad issue. Any change of any parameter located in the acceptable range should be examined in terms of its impact on the results obtained—brightness in the simplest form, classification results in an advanced form. Therefore, in addition to the above-discussed impact of the size, position and rotation of the *ROI* on the obtained results of the mean brightness, it is also interesting to analyse the impact of lighting or positioning the pattern relative to the analysed object. It is possible to analyse independently the sensitivity of the classification results to repositioning and resizing the *ROI* and the impact of noise in the image (due to both the properties of the camera and the type and brightness of lighting). Below there are the results of measurement of *ACC* for the manually selected *ROIs*, with the test area being moved in the row axis by $\Delta m = \pm 20$ pixels and in the column axis by $\Delta n = \pm 20$ pixels. Two features are analysed: the mean brightness in the *ROI* and the standard deviation of the mean. The results obtained are shown in Figs. 6.6 and 6.7.

The source code in this case is a bit different than that presented in the previous subchapters, i.e.:

```
L1=load(['D:/k/_I20_L0-511_13-1-
2016_13.5.59.cube',mat2str(80),'.mat']);
Lgrayi=mat2gray(L1.L1);
figure; res=[];        hObj=waitbar(0,'Please wait...');
[X,Y,I,RECTP] = IMCROP(Lgrayi);
for deltam=-20:20
    RECTT=RECTP;
    RECTT(2)=RECTT(2)+deltam;
    meas=[];
    measT=[];
    for i=1:128
        L1=load(['D:/k/_I20_L0-511_13-1-
2016_13.5.59.cube',mat2str(i),'.mat']);
        Lgrayi=mat2gray(L1.L1);
        LgrayiP=IMCROP(Lgrayi,RECTP);
        LgrayiT=IMCROP(Lgrayi,RECTT);
        meas(i,1)=mean(LgrayiP(:));
        meas(i,2)=std(LgrayiP(:));
        measT(i,1)=mean(LgrayiT(:));
        measT(i,2)=std(LgrayiT(:));
    end
    TRR=zeros([size(meas,1), 1]);
    TRR(20:110)=1;
    species=[];
    for ijj=1:length(TRR)
        if TRR(ijj)==1
            species{ijj}='Yes';
        else
            species{ijj}='No';
        end
    end
    svmStruct = svmtrain(meas,species');
    grpname = svmclassify(svmStruct,measT);
    TP=sum( strcmp(grpname,'Yes').*
strcmp(species','Yes') );
    TN=sum( strcmp(grpname,'No')  .*
strcmp(species','No')  );
    FN=sum( strcmp(grpname,'No')  .*
strcmp(species','Yes')  );
    FP=sum( strcmp(grpname,'Yes').*
strcmp(species','No')  );
    ACC= round((TP+TN)/(FN+FP+TN+TP).*100);
    TPR= round(TP/(TP+FN).*100);
    SPC= round(TN/(TN+FP).*100);
    res=[res;[deltam, TP, TN, FN, FP, ACC, TPR, SPC]];
    waitbar((deltam+20)/40)
end
```

```
    close(hObj)
figure; plot(res(:,1),res(:,6),'-r*'); hold on; grid
on;
xlabel('\Delta m
[pixel]','FontSize',14,'FontAngle','Italic')
ylabel('ACC [%]','FontSize',14,'FontAngle','Italic')
```

The source code in its first part enables to manually identify the *ROI* in the image for $i = 80$. Then the test *ROI* is artificially moved, i.e.: RECTT = RECTP; RECTT (2) = RECTT(2) + deltam; and two features are calculated: the mean brightness mean(LgrayiP(:)) and the standard deviation of the mean std (LgrayiP(:). The length of the training and test vectors is the same and is equal to the total number of frames, i.e. $I = 128$. In the next stage, the SVM classifier is trained (variable meas) and tested, and *ACC* is calculated (variable measT). The results are shown in the last part of the presented source code figure; plot...).

Noise can be introduced artificially to the *i*th sequence of images using the previously applied function imnoise. In this case, the value of *ACC* for the SVM classifier (as in the previous example) was initially analysed for different values of variance $v \in (0, 1)$ and a zero mean value. The results obtained are shown in Fig. 6.8.

The form of the source code is almost identical to the previous example. The only significant difference is the change in the value of v in each loop circulation in the

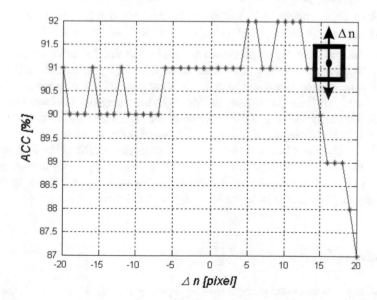

Fig. 6.7 Graph of changes in *ACC* for different values of *Δn*

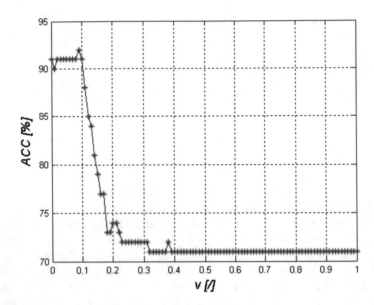

Fig. 6.8 Graph of changes in *ACC* for different values of *v*

range from 0 to 1 every 0.01 and the notation `LgraiTm = imnoise(IMCROP`
`(Lgrayi,RECTT), 'gaussian',0,v)` allowing for the addition of noise to the
image. Only one type of noise (`'gaussian'`) is analysed. By a slight modification of
the source code, similar tests can be performed for the following noise types:
`'localvar'`, `'poisson'`, `'salt & pepper'` or `'speckle'`.

It is apparent from the graph presented in Fig. 6.8 that the value of accuracy is
reduced for successive values of variance from 92 to 72%—by exactly 20%. This is
a significant change when compared, for example, with the graphs shown in
Figs. 6.6 and 6.7. For repositioning the test *ROI*, the change in *ACC* was only a few
per cent. This information gives the picture of the algorithm sensitivity (in this case
the results of SVM classification) to the degree of noise in the image.

At the end it should be emphasized that the presented results of the evaluation of
the algorithm sensitivity to parameter changes are exemplary. They do not exhaust
in any way the full diversity of hyperspectral images dependent on individual
variability of patients, the imaging area, lighting and many others.

References

1. KOPROWSKI R.: *Quantitative assessment of the impact of biomedical image acquisition on the results obtained from image analysis and processing.* BioMedical Engineering OnLine 2014, 13:93.

2. Gonzalez R, Woods R: Digital Image Processing. New York: Addison-Wesley Publishing Company; 1992.
3. Sonka M, Michael Fitzpatrick J: Medical Image Processing and Analysis. In Handbook of Medical, Imaging. Belligham: SPIE; 2000.
4. Dash M, Liu H: Feature Selection for Classification, in Intelligent Data Analysis. New York: Elsevier; 1997:131–156.
5. Duda R, Hart P, Stork D: Reference Classification. 2nd edition. New York: John Wiley & Sons, Inc.; 2001.

Chapter 7
Conclusions

This monograph presents both new and known methods of analysis and processing of hyperspectral medical images. The developed GUI allows for easy and intuitive performance of basic operations both on a single image and a sequence of hyperspectral images. These are operations such as filtration, separation of an object, measurements of basic and complex texture features as well as classification. Therefore the developed GUI may be useful both diagnostically in the analysis, for example, of dermatological images and may also serve as a foundation for software development. In addition, the monograph presents new approaches to analysis and processing of hyperspectral images. After minor modifications, they can be used for other purposes and image analyses. The algorithm sensitivity to changes in the selected parameters has also been evaluated. The presented source code can be used without licensing restrictions provided this monograph is cited. It should also be emphasized here that the author is not responsible for the consequences of wrong use and operation of this software. Despite the author's best efforts, errors may occur in the presented source code. The presented software is deliberately free of restrictions, which should encourage the reader to its subsequent modifications and improvements. An equally open issue is the time optimization of the described methods of image analysis and processing, which has been deliberately omitted in almost the entire monograph (except Table 4.1). Thus the presented software does not close the interesting subject of analysis and processing of hyperspectral medical images.

© Springer International Publishing AG 2017   123
R. Koprowski, *Processing of Hyperspectral Medical Images*,
Studies in Computational Intelligence 682,
DOI 10.1007/978-3-319-50490-2_7

Appendix

A set of Matlab *m-files* is attached to this monograph so that the reader does not have to rewrite each selected part of the source code from the text. According to the information given in the monograph, the files have been divided into two containers:

- *GUI_ver_pre.zip*—containing 5 *m-files* enabling to test the initial version of the application;
- *GUI_ver_full.zip*—containing 21 test *m-files* and 15 GUI files.

The container *GUI_ver_pre.zip* includes 5 *m-files* with the following names and functionalities:

- read_envi_header—reading the header from *.hdr* file,
- read_envi_data—reading data from *.cube, *.raw* or *.dat* files,
- GUI_hyperspectral_trans—affine transformations of the image,
- GUI_hyperspectral—main GUI file (run first),
- GUI_hyperspectral_fun—function responsible for the functionality of individual menu elements.

The container *GUI_ver_full.zip* includes 36 *m-files* (including *m-files* for tests) with the following names and functionalities:

- read_envi_header—reading the header from *.hdr* file (the same as in the container *GUI_ver_pre.zip*)
- read_envi_data—reading data from *.cube, *.raw* or *.dat* files (the same as in the container *GUI_ver_pre.zip*)
- GUI_hyperspectral_trans—affine transformations of the image (the same as in the container *GUI_ver_pre.zip*)
- GUI_hyperspectral—main GUI file extended with respect to the file from the container *GUI_ver_pre.zip* (run first),

© Springer International Publishing AG 2017
R. Koprowski, *Processing of Hyperspectral Medical Images*,
Studies in Computational Intelligence 682,
DOI 10.1007/978-3-319-50490-2

- `GUI_hyperspectral_fun`—function responsible for the functionality of individual menu elements extended with respect to the file from the container *GUI_ver_pre.zip*,
- `Class_test`—*m-file* for testing different classification variants,
- `Class_test2`—*m-file* for testing different classification variants,
- `Class_test3`—*m-file* for testing different classification variants,
- `Class_test4`—*m-file* for testing different classification variants,
- `Class_test5`—*m-file* for testing different classification variants,
- `Gauss_test`—*m-file* for testing different variants of the Gaussian function,
- `Gauss_test2`—*m-file* for testing different variants of the Gaussian function,
- `Gauss_test3`—*m-file* for testing different variants of the Gaussian function,
- `Gauss_test4`—*m-file* for testing different variants of the Gaussian function,
- `Dergauss`—function of the Gaussian function derivatives,
- `GUI_hyperspectral_adaptive_filter`—function of the adaptive filter,
- `GUI_hyperspectral_class`—function of selecting classification type,
- `GUI_hyperspectral_class_dec_tree`—classifier function—decision trees,
- `GUI_hyperspectral_class_disc`—classifier function—discriminant analysis,
- `GUI_hyperspectral_naive_bayes`—classifier function—naive Bayes classifier,
- `GUI_hyperspectral_class_svm`—classifier function—SVM,
- `GUI_hyperspectral_diff`—function responsible for calculating brightness differences,
- `GUI_hyperspectral_dilate_c`—function of conditional dilation,
- `GUI_hyperspectral_erode_c`—function of conditional erosion,
- `GUI_hyperspectral_erode_dilate_test`—*m-file* for testing the properties of conditional erosion and dilation,
- `GUI_hyperspectral_erode_dilate_test2`—*m-file* for testing the properties of conditional erosion and dilation,
- `GUI_hyperspectral_erode_dilate_test3`—*m-file* for testing the properties of conditional erosion and dilation,
- `GUI_hyperspectral_erode_dilate_test4`—*m-file* for testing the properties of conditional erosion and dilation,
- `GUI_hyperspectral_filter_test`—*m-file* for testing dedicated filtration,
- `GUI_hyperspectral_filter_test2`—*m-file* for testing dedicated filtration,

- GUI_hyperspectral_qtdecomp_test—*m-file* for testing square-tree decomposition,
- GUI_hyperspectral_qtdecomp_test2—*m-file* for testing square-tree decomposition,
- GUI_hyperspectral_para_change—*m-file* for testing the effect of parameter changes on the results obtained,
- GUI_hyperspectral_para_changes2—*m-file* for testing the effect of parameter changes on the results obtained,
- GUI_hyperspectral_para_changes3—*m-file* for testing the effect of parameter changes on the results obtained,
- GUI_hyperspectral_para_changes4—*m-file* for testing the effect of parameter changes on the results obtained.

The two described containers containing all the *m-files* discussed in this monograph along with the source codes are available at http://extras.springer.com/.

Printed in the United States
By Bookmasters